# *What is* COLOR BLINDNESS?



## *What to Know if You're Diagnosed With Color Blindness*

Egill Hansen

Originally published in Norwegian as Fargeblindhet, First Edition 2010,
Gyldendal Norsk Forlag


ISBN: 1492201162
ISBN-13: 9781492201168

# ACKNOWLEDGEMENTS

I would like to thank John McKee for reading through and correcting the language in the English version. I thank Constance Hale for help in editing and improving the language. I also thank Geir Qvale for computer service and preparing the pictures. Finally I thank my daughter Marianne and my son Morten for valuable assistance.

# CONTENTS

# PREFACE

In 1992 a 21-year-old man eager for advancement in the military came to me for a consultation. I will call him Thor. When he was 9 or 10, a school doctor had found that he had a red-green color deficiency, which an older brother also had. (Two other brothers had normal color vision.) This had not compromised his achievement either in school or in work. At the time Thor came to see me, he was working successfully as a milling operator at a weapons factory, but color blindness was disqualifying him for advancement in the military weaponry field. He had seen an ophthalmologist, who referred him to me for diagnosis.

I was a head physician of ophthalmology at the National Hospital and specialized in color blindness. Thor was one of some thousands patients I saw in a career that spanned three decades. Like Thor, about eight percent of all men have a weakness in red-green color perception (and fewer than 0.5 percent of women), many people remain unaware of their own limited perception of color or of how color blindness affects the people around them.

This book is written for those who want to know more.

First, there are those who are simply interested in knowing more about various genetic conditions. Then there are those whose curiosity has been aroused because of contact with color blind people in their families, workplaces, or schools. Some readers—psychologists, teachers, vocational-rehabilitation specialists—may need tangible information so as better to serve clients and patients. Some may work within the health care system, where they are eager to be able to quickly identify color vision problems in order to help their patients.

Some readers may be physicians who are directly responsible for regularly checking color vision, whether school doctors, company doctors, merchant marine doctors, military doctors, doctors for pilots and train conductors, ophthalmologists specializing in acquired visual defects, and optometrists helping patients enhance their vision through glasses and contact lenses. (Principles of color-vision tests are mentioned here, though practical guidance for the use of the tests is outside the purview of this book.)

Then, of course, there are those for whom some form of color blindness has meant that they couldn't make their best art, do their best job, or advance in a line of work they are otherwise well suited to.

This book will provide basic facts about defects in color vision—how they arise, how they become apparent, how many different types occur, and which diagnostic methods are used. I will touch on some theoretical data, but this book is not intended to cover all what we in the medical profession have discovered over the past 300 years. I have attempted to include the most important information and will refer to other resources where those seeking more exhaustive answers can find them. You can read the chapters separately or together, with some information included in more than one place.

I hope that whether you are reading this book because color blindness has touched you, or because you are simply interested in learning more about medical conditions, you will find it as fascinating as I have over my long career.

# I: THE EXTENT OF COLOR BLINDNESS

# CHAPTER 1: THE CLASSIC STORY

Let us return to Thor, the patient who came to me eager to enter a military career. After Thor told me about being diagnosed in school and sharing this condition with one of his three brothers, I asked him how he experienced his condition. He told me that he had trouble noticing bright colors, especially pale red and pale green. He had discovered that when out picking berries with friends, he had trouble sorting strawberries and red cowberries, while the red-orange cloudberries and red rowanberries stood out. When looking out to the sea at night, Thor couldn't tell which side of a boat was turned toward him, as the red lanterns on the port side and the green lanterns on the starboard side looked identical to him. When driving, he had no difficulty seeing red and green traffic lights, but he had been surprised once when a large green warning sign he saw from afar turned out to be red when he stopped beneath it.

Thor had been a good student and had not felt handicapped at work. He had operated a machine at a weapons factory for many years and wanted to use his technical background for further education in the military. But regulations prohibited someone with his history of red-green color deficiency from entering officer candidate school.

My examination revealed that he had a red-green color-vision deficiency of a marked degree, which we in the field call deuteranopia ("green blindness"). Although he had never felt impeded by this condition, it was indeed severe enough to stop his military career.

Thor's experience illustrates several different factors important to anyone interested in color blindness. First, color blindness is a hereditary trait, confirmed in this case by the fact that Thor had a brother who shared the condition. Second, Thor's difficulties were consistent with the commonest form of color-vision deficiency, namely a red-green deficiency. Third, even with this high-degree of color-vision defect, Thor had been little troubled by his color-vision deficiency and had successfully worked in a branch of weapons production. Fourth, his condition would indeed restrict his ability to train further in such a specialized branch of the military.

There are two final and important points: varying degrees of congenital red-green color-vision deficiency are found in one out of every 12 men. But without close medical examination, people like Thor can go through life without basic knowledge of the degree or type of their own color vision. (The incidence in women is far lower: about 1 in 220 women have the same type of color-vision deficiency.)

## WHAT IS COLOR BLINDNESS?

> Color blindness means the inability or reduced ability to see colors *in the usual way*. It includes the inability to differentiate between color hues, so that the colors can be confused with each other. It may manifest so that a person cannot recognize colors when they appear in natural surroundings.

Sometimes one can be surprised by other persons' opinion of colors. Some divergence is within what is to be expected between individuals. But in other cases the divergence might be greater. Discrimination of colors and their recognition can be problematic where other persons have no problems.

From a medical perspective, the ability to "see" colors means to be able to differentiate among them and to distinguish colors from black, white, and gray. This ability is not vital. Yet color vision allows visual nuance and a richness of perception in the world around us. This nuance and richness might be sublime—the fall colors on a Vermont mountainside in October, perhaps, or the beautiful blues of the sea off a Caribbean island. But they might also be mundane—the small tablets in a pill organizer, for example, or the coffee cups on a shelf in Crate and Barrel.

Color blindness is really a misnomer; it does not exclusively refer to a black-and-white world. It is used as a general term for all degrees and types of deviant color vision. The term is also used for minor color deficiencies where colors usually can be seen and separated, and in cases where there are uncertainty, if at all, may apply to weak chromatic colors only (like pink and peach). But it could also apply to severe color deficiency with great uncertainty even for bright colors of good saturation (like the red color of a fire engine).

For people with deficient color vision some colors seem dull and difficult to identify. They could be similar to shades of gray. A poor perception of colors of this type does not concern all colors, but only *certain* color tints or hues. At the same time other hues can be seen clearly (and here the term "color blind" is not appropriate).

Confronted with the colors he sees as pale or gray areas in the color circle , the color deficient person will not have any information of the hues, but *the brightness* of colors can still be perceived. Therefore one is not really "blind" completely for those colors either. The critical colors which are unsaturated and approach gray, can easily be confused with each other. Such confusions are characteristic for each type of color deficiency and they follow a certain pattern. Color blindness is accordingly not a good and complete term, as it is widely used for a great variety of types and degrees.

The main characteristic of strong color blindness is difficulty with red and green. That would suggest that all the colors in the spectrum would fall into a yellow and a blue zone. Do the color blinds see the world in only yellow and blue? No. They believe they experience red and green as well. However, they can have great difficulties in *identifying* red and green colors, especially with colors of poor saturation. A certain instability in their identification of colors is sometimes reported by the color blind. A dull brown sheet of paper—much like a shopping bag at an average supermarket—is sometimes called green, another time brown and a third time red by the same person. Likewise it may occur that gray colors are seen as colored, partly as red and partly as green or brown. Blurred yellow colors are often believed to be green.

Blue-yellow color blindness, which is mostly an acquired defect (from accidents or diseases), can entail confusion of blue with green and violet with yellow-green. To some with blue-yellow color blindness, yellow is an invisible color: they cannot see marks or letters written with a yellow pencil on white paper.

Color blindness can be of different degrees—from exceptionally mild to pronounced. The different degrees do matter and should be tested for.

Most people who have color-vision deficiencies are in a mild or moderate group. They don't experience faults worth mentioning in their color vision. They distinguish red and green colors, and they find the right colors in the paintbox. Still their weakness can be revealed when they are confronted with colors of weak saturation or by a fast change in colors, as when a warning light changes from red to yellow. There can be a tendency also for people with slightly affected color-vision deficiency to mistake certain colors under unfavorable conditions (as in rain or fog).

Out in nature the various kinds of color blindness become quite striking when a number of subjects are asked to identify different kinds of berries, and especially strawberries which are usually overlooked by people with color vision deficiencies. However, a so-called "red blind" person can most often see strawberries—they look very dark to him. On the contrary, he could hardly find cloudberries, the attractive orange berries growing in the mountains. Cowberries, the more common red berries in the woods, may be difficult to see both for people who are "red weak" and those who are "green weak." Some color blind people say that they cannot see cowberries at a distance when other people may see lots of berries in the same location. However, when they come close, they too can see the berries. A "green blind" man could hardly see ripe cloudberries while he could easily see unripe berries.

Another man, John, had difficulty seeing the difference between brown and green, also at short distance. He could not see strawberries at a distance even when others pointed them out to him, but he saw them when up close. He identified colors best after focusing on the objects for a while, but in his perception the colors could change character, and his identification could be influenced by the opinion of others, especially when the colors under question were yellow and green.

A "color-weak" man, Jim, had difficulties especially with pale colors as when he could hardly distinguish between yellow and orange. Seeing the difference between the colors yellow, green and red at a distance was difficult. Likewise, he had experienced increased difficulty with colors in hazy weather.

## HOW IS COLOR BLINDNESS DISCOVERED?

Practical situations offer clues. One clue is when a person names a color differently from others. Another clue is when one person believes that colors are being misidentified by others—or in a book, catalog, or box of crayons. Yet another is if, when shown an obvious palette of colors, one person cannot tell one color (for example yellow- green) from another (like, red- orange). Others experience no problems with this task, but they can become uncomfortable when being confronted with certain color contrasts. Appropriate tests can determine whether the color vision is normal or deviant.

The most important moment for discovering color blindness is a child's first months at school. I met one boy, age 7 whom I shall call Tommy, who had trouble on his first days of classes. Although he didn't yet know it, he had a "green blind" type of color vision deficiency, in which chiefly colors from green to red purple were confused. During a drawing lesson, he wanted to add grass and leaves to his picture, but he used brown instead of dark green. (Other children with the green blind deficiency might confuse dark-red, green, brown and light-brown, and still others might confuse violet with blue). Color blindness can sometimes be masked by compensation or coping strategies. Some children rely on other kids to pick out the right colors for them. In the case of Tommy, his father had marked off the pencils in his kit

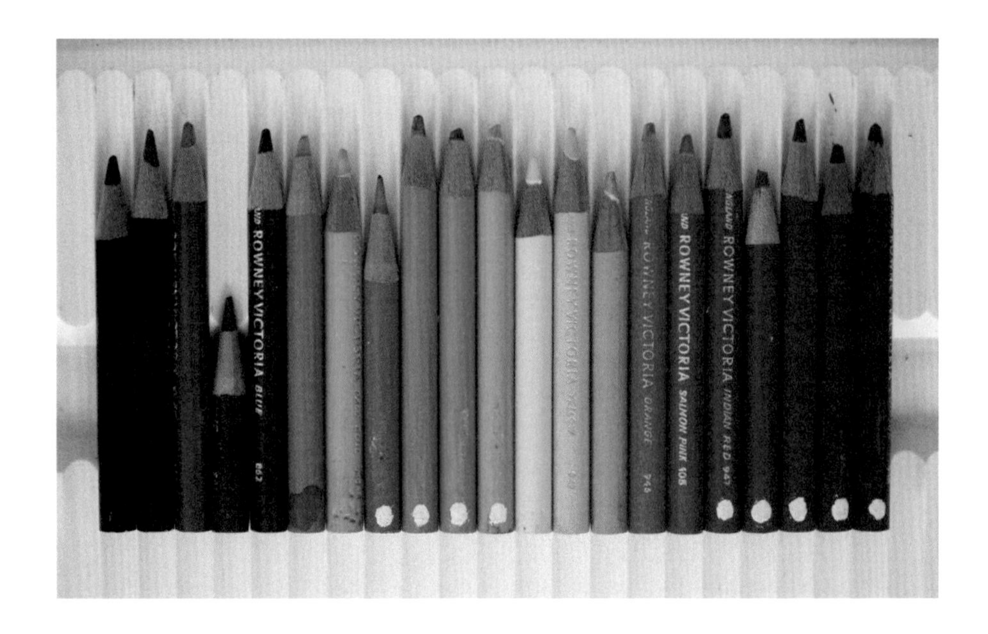


Figure 1. From the paint box of Tommy, a boy in his first year in school. His father added white dots to each of the colored pencils whose shade he could not differentiate.

so that the doctor and teacher could see which colors he usually confused (see figure 1).

A 29 year old man, Simon, who visited me, told he had suspected that something was wrong with his color vision in elementary school, but he assumed that it was because he had not "learned" the proper names of colors. At that time, of course, he had no idea that he was color blind. As an adult, though, he began to have inklings. He grew up to be a car dealer and had once referred to a beige car as green. On another occasion, he had correctly noticed that a car that had been repainted, had received the wrong shade of paint. Interestingly, his co-workers did not even see the change at first but later agreed that there was a real difference in shades. The color in question was a brown metallic with a slight element of grayish blue ("silver fox"). In this case, the "green blind" man had a sharper eye for differences in color shades than others. My examination revealed that he had a color deficiency called "deuteranopia" or green blindness.

A journalist, called Ola, came to me last year in order to find out the diagnosis of his color vision defect. His story is related in *"My Life as a Color Blind"* - an interview-article in the newspaper's magazine (Henmo 2010). He writes that fresh grass appeared orange to him. An orange football on the grass was invisible. When his wife enthusiastically described the crackling red flowers of a hibiscus, he only saw green leaves. I examined him and diagnosed him with a protanopic type of deficiency, or "red blindness". He told an amusing story from a soccer game where his favorite team was playing in green costumes and the competitors in orange: "It was highly confusing. Twenty men in the same costumes were running aimlessly between two keepers. Some defense players hurled the ball toward their own goal. The team members tackled each other violently and hard. The referee blew randomly for offside, free kicks, corner and goals."

Color blinds are not a homogeneous group but comprise individuals of great variation. Even if it were possible to find individuals with exactly the same defect, the attitude to colors and their feeling of colors would be quite different (as reported by R W Pickford in the book *"Individual Differences in Color Vision"* (Pickford 1951). Some people are aware that they perceive color differently from friends, family, or colleagues. Others may not have noticed any difference at all and may be surprised when a color vision test reveals deficiency.

One of the serious challenges in research into color blindness is that it is difficult for the non color blind to understand how the world is perceived by the color blind and vice versa. To make matters worse, the colors used on test charts in consultation rooms are typically difficult to distinguish and can lead to unfortunate miscommunications between patient and doctor.

Yet, it is critically important that even slight degrees of color-vision deficiencies are discovered, since color blindness can be relevant in occupations that demand quick recognition of colors. This applies especially to red and green signals used in communication and safety systems for land, sea, and air travel.

An ideal best method for studying color blindness would be to study a subject who has one eye color blind and the other normal. In some extremely rare cases, such persons have been found. The heredity researcher H. Kalmus, in his 1965 book *Diagnosis and Genetics of Defective Colour Vision*, wrote about a young woman who had normal color vision in her right eye, but was "green blind" in her left eye. When seeing with both eyes, she had a complete color experience and could name colors adequately. When she closed the right eye, all red and green had gone, and her color perception was limited to grey, yellow, and blue. From her description we can have a precise knowledge of what color blindness involves.

# CHAPTER 2:
# HISTORIC NOTES

Colors have had symbolic value throughout history. Certain colors have special meaning. Flags and banners in bright colors have a special appeal. They have been used to stand in for neighborhoods in Siena and for nations as disparate as Spain and Samoa. Leonardo da Vinci (1452-1519) was engaged in dealing with colors. He defined four "simple colors": red, green, yellow and blue—along with white and black.

In a maritime context, red and green have long been used to indicate the sides of the ship: red for the port side and green for starboard. In fact, it was at sea that it was first noticed how some people were unable to distinguish the lanterns in the darkness, thus rendering them unable to decide the course of the ship. It was clear that some sailors were "blind" to colors.

Accounts of irregularities in color vision, oddly enough, appeared rather late in the medical professional field. Professor W. Jaeger in Heidelberg, produced a comprehensive survey of color vision research with the key to the information of the different kinds of congenital red-green disturbances (Jaeger 1994).

## KEY SCIENTISTS

One of the first people to mention red-green color-vision deficiency in a scientific article was Joseph Huddart, an $18^{th}$-century sea captain and hydrographer whose description of three brothers of a Quaker family in Britain "who could not distinguish Colours" was entered into the proceedings of the Royal Society in London in 1777. (Other, less precise accounts had also been reported earlier.)

Also in 1777, George Palmer, a glass dealer with an interest in colors, suggested that the retina contained three types of fibers corresponding to three physical types of light; an account which was called attention to by Mollon (Mollon 1997). This physiological hypothesis is today recognized as the modern theory of trichromasy (even though Palmer's did not withstand scrutiny).

Palmer's hypothesis was published 25 years before a famous lecture by the English scientist Thomas Young. In addition to making notable contributions to the fields of light, solid mechanics, energy, physiology, language, musical harmony, and Egyptology, Young postulated in 1802 three types of color receptors in the normal eye. This theory formed the base of the most appropriate explanation of the deficiencies of color vision. (The theory is now known and accepted as the Young-Helmholtz theory.)

John Dalton (1766-1844), the famous English chemist, physicist and founder of modern atomic theory, gave a vivid description of his own color blindness in a 1794 paper, "Extraordinary facts relating to the vision of colours": He reported that to him, lips, a rose, and the sky were similar in color. Grass and sealing wax, also, appeared the same color to him. Dalton concluded that "the part of the picture which others call red, looks to me to be only a shade or a defect in the light." Orange, yellow, and green, he added "are what I would call different tints of yellow."

*Many English protested Dalton's name being connected to color deficiency. (Dalton himself didn't give much credence to the honor.) In the search for good terms for the condition, "disease" and "illness" were often used, and people affected were even called "color cripples." "Color blindness" was eventually proposed as a term and was accepted, except in France, where "Daltonism" is still the common name* (Breslauer Zeitung 1878).

From Dalton color blindness was called "Daltonism", a term also used today.

Dalton himself had the theory that his condition was a result of blue—rather than clear—liquid in his eye. This, he theorized, obstructed the red light. He decided that his eyes should be examined after his death by his assistant Joseph Ransom. The autopsy was done after Dalton's death on July 27, 1844. The liquid in Dalton's eyes was clear so could not explain his color deficiency. However, the puzzle was solved more recently by a DNA analysis (parts of his eyes had been kept by the Manchester Literary and Philosophical Society.) The scientist D.M. Hunt, along with colleagues at the University of London, revealed in 1995 that Dalton had the condition called deuteranopia (green blindness) (Hunt 1995).

"Daltoniana" has been chosen as the name of the regular newsletters edited by the International Colour Vision Society, an association for research especially on color-vision deficiencies.

Johann Wolfgang Goethe (1749 - 1832), the great German Poet, presented his own color theory. (His interest in the nature of colors rivaling his interest in literature.) Among Goethe's practical experiments was one in which he presented colored slips of paper to his subjects. When they identified yellow and green slips as similar to orange, and red-purple as matching purple and blue, Goethe erroneously called this "blue blindness", while in reality this kind of mistakes is a characteristic of red-green blindness. (Jaeger 1994).

## SEMINAL TESTS

The physicist August Seebeck, whose father was a friend of Goethe, described two types of red-green deficiency, one type seeing the spectrum shortened in the long wavelength (red) end and the other seeing the spectrum in full length. He so realized that there were two types of red-green-blindness.

In 1881, Lord Rayleigh discovered that mixtures of red and green spectral lights could be adjusted so as to make them appear identical with a yellow light in the spectrum. Most people with a normal color vision could do the matches within narrow limits. Interestingly, some people mixed in an abundance of red, while others added too much green when matching the yellow light. They revealed incomplete forms of color blindness, which were designated *protanomaly* and *deuteranomaly* respectively. Based on the same principle an instrument for the exact classification of all types of red-green deficiency was introduced by W. A. Nagel in 1907.

Gradually, there was agreement that normal color vision included three components of which one component was missing in the color blind. J. von Kries in 1911 suggested the term *protanopia* for complete "red blindness," *deuteranopia* for complete "green blindness," and *tritanopia* for complete "blue blindness." Those are the terms used today, and they indicate whether a person is missing the first, second or third color mechanism. Missing the first mechanism causes a protanopic defect, the second mechanism a deuteranopic defect and the third a tritanopic color defect.

After a number of great but somewhat mysterious railway accidents at the end of the 19th century, deficient color vision was suspected as a possible cause. Soon color- vision testing of engine drivers began. Tests using the different-colored light from lanterns had been used in England since 1853, when the Great North Railway Company decided on a new standard for color vision in railway transport and later on also for maritime transport. The same tests were introduced in France in about 1858.

One of the first generally accessible tests to point out color blindness was the Holmgren wool test, first used in 1869 by the Swedish physiologist Frithiof Holmgren (1831-1897). Holmgren suspected that the engineer of a train in a well-publicized railway accident at Lagerlunda, Sweden, suffered from color blindness. He set out to test this theory by examining employees of the Uppsala-Gøteborg railroad company. The Holmgren wool test contained a collection of differently colored skeins of wool. An examinee would be presented with one wool skein out of a collection of more than 100 differently colored ones and asked to find other samples of the same color. Many strange proposals might result if the examinee had a color-vision deficiency. The test was not standardized, and sometimes the examiner could be quite as confused as the examinee. Nevertheless this test was the preferred test for many doctors up to modern times. The test, however, is only of historic interest; it is not in use today.

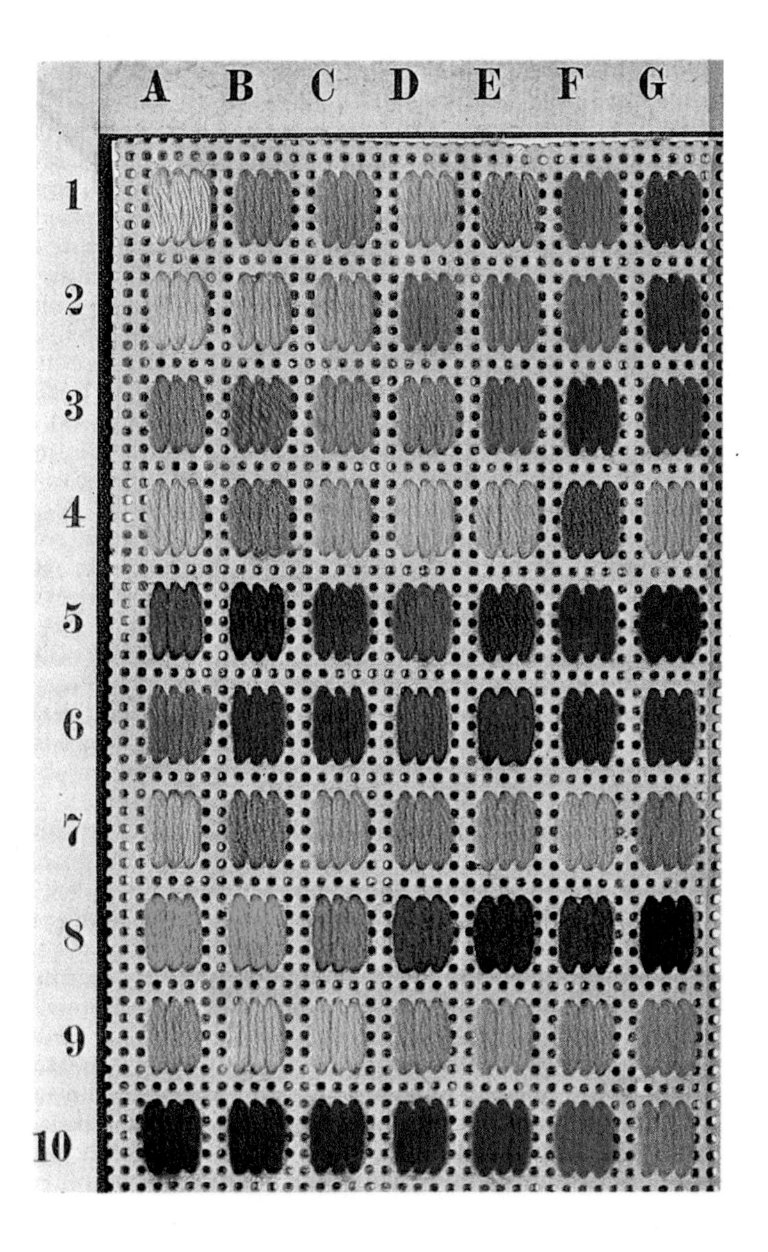


Figure 2. Daae's test table for the examination of the color blind (Berlin 1878). Approximately similar colors are shown in two rows, number 8 (green) and number 10 (red). Stating more than these two rows as having similar colors indicates color blindness.

A somewhat more standardized test, also like Holmgren's test being based on wool patches, was introduced by Anders Daae, a general practitioner in Kragerø, Norway, in 1877 and in Germany in 1878 (Daae 1877). In this, differently colored patches of wool were arranged on a grid in fixed order. The colors in each row were all different except in two rows where the colors were similar for all patches[1]. Among 10 rows of colors the examinee was asked to point out the rows with identical colors. Stating more than two rows with similar colors indicated color blindness (Figure 2). It is told that Daae in Kragerø veritably chased color blind people, especially sailors. There was great excitement among the sailors when he did find someone who could not discriminate the colors of the ship's lanterns from each other.

The test was well received and in Germany ranked (by Cohn) second to Holmgren's test, and surpassing Stilling's test which also appeared in 1878.

In 1878 Professor Hermann Cohn in Breslau was engaged in finding better color vision tests (Cohn 1878). While his investigations were going on he received the table made by Daae in Kragerø. He pronounced it "ausgezeichnet" (excellent).

The Stilling test was constructed by German ophthalmologist Jacob Stilling, who was a professor at the University of Strasbourg (Stilling 1878). The design of the test charts followed a new idea based on colors which were commonly confused by color defective persons. Stilling had some color blind painters making a palette consisting of colors which to them looked identical, however, looking clearly different to people with normal color vision. He constructed figures against backgrounds, both in colors confused by the color defectives. The figures were then invisible to a color blind person, but were distinct to normal persons. Accordingly, there was no need to name the colors, but only to identify the figures. (It can thus be stated that the color sense had been "translated" to the sphere of form sense). This test was far more suitable to point out color-vision deficiency than the tests known until then.

1 Concerning the production of the test Daae's contemporary friend Bundi considered that his sister - Sofie - who had a broderie shop in the town, mounted the colors.

It is interesting to read the Cohn's review of the Stilling test (Cohn 1878): "Without doubt many color blind are unable to read the charts in the Stilling test, but not all. On the other hand too many are diagnosed as color blind by the Stilling charts. It appears that a great number of intelligent (!) people who name every color placed before them correctly and arrange the wool samples satisfactorily are completely unable to read the letters. Even highly educated persons have commented on the colors selected for the green-blind: "Such strange colors I cannot name."

However, paradoxically, Stilling's test was not well received when it appeared in Germany in 1878.

At that time, mild degrees of color blindness were largely unrecognized. The Stilling test was the forerunner of other tests based on the same principle, of pseudo-isochromatic design which are the most commonly used tests for diagnosing color deficiencies today. Among these the best known is the test introduced by the Japanese Dr. Shinobu Ishihara in 1916. Color-vision tests were used more enthusiastically in Japan than elsewhere, and neither in any other countries were so many people denied trade and education because of color blindness.

# CHAPTER 3: TYPES AND DEGREES OF COLOR DEFICIENCIES

One differentiates between congenital and acquired color deficiencies. The first group is hereditary and is due to wrong pigments in the retinal receptors. The last group is caused by disease processes or damage in the visual apparatus (chapter 5).

## CONGENITAL COLOR DEFICIENCIES

Most commonly seen are the red-green color deficiencies which occur in about 8 per cent of the male population and about 0.4 per cent in women.

Red-green color deficiencies are classified as:

*Protanopia (P) "**red blindness**" and *Protanomaly (PA) "**red weakness**".

Collective term: Protan defects (P+PA). The fundamental failure is loss of perception of long wavelength light.

*Deuteranopia (D) "**green blindness**" and *Deuteranomaly (DA) "**green weakness**".

Collective term: Deutan defects (D+DA). The fundamental failure is loss of perception of middle wavelength light.

Blue-yellow color deficiencies are classified as :

*Tritanopia (T) "**blue blindness**" and Tritanomaly (TA) "**blue weakness**".

Collective term: Tritan defects (T+TA). The fundamental failure is loss of perception of short wavelength light.

Types of color vision consist in separate groups:

* **Trichromatic vision** (normal) requires lights from three different wavelengths in the spectrum to obtain a match with a random color.

* **Anomal trichromacy** (PA, DA, TA) requires lights from three different wavelengths in the spectrum to obtain a match with a random color, but in disproportionate amount. Anomaleous trichromacy includes protanomaly, deuteranomaly and tritanomaly.

***Dichromacy (P, D, T)** requires lights from only two different wavelengths in the spectrum to obtain a match with a random color. Dichromacy includes protanopia, deuteranopia and tritanopia.

***Monochromacy** (total color blindness) needs light from any wavelength in the spectrum to match a random color.

In men, 5 per cent are deuteranomaleous, 1 per cent are deuteranopes, 1 per cent are protanomaleous and 1 per cent are protanopes according to Georg Waaler (Waaler 1927) in his book about the hereditary relationship of congenital red-green blindness[2].

Congenital blue blindness (tritanopia and tritanomaly) are very seldom found (Kalmus 1965). Kalmus estimated the occurrence between 1:13.000 and 1:65.000. Also total color blindness is diagnosed very seldom, in about 1:72,000 (The Norwegian Registry of Blindness 1995).

In particular Waaler's data are very accurate. He examined more than 18.000 school children in Oslo, half of them boys and half girls. He studied in detail whether the number of the color blind he had found in the boys agreed with his expectations of the occurrence in the girls. As 8.01 per cent of the men had a red-green color vision deficiency, he expected about 0.64 per cent to be found in women, but still he found only 0.44 per cent. And this discrepancy, as we shall see, led to the explanation that the genes for red-green color deficiency are localized in two different places.

Color blindness occurs in many degrees. It is appropriate to differentiate between color blindness of **mild** degree, **moderate** degree and **pronounced** degree. In addition a separate group of color defects of **especially mild** degree (minimal color vision deficiency) should be included.

The type of deficiency may indicate the degree of color deficiency. However, many exceptions can be seen. In particular, there are great variations among the anomalous trichromats, varying from serious defects to very light defects. Likewise, the dichromats may be quite different in their ability to master color vision tasks. More accurately the degree of color deficiency can be determined by the use of a battery of different tests.

Most people who are color deficient are in the two first groups - mild and moderate degrees. They don't experience faults worth mentioning in their color vision. They distinguish red and green colors, and they find the right

---

2 The exact figures found by Waaler were: 5,06 per cent deuteranomaleous, 1,03 per cent deuteranopes, 1,04 per cent protanomaleous and 0,88 per cent protanopes.

colors in the paint box. Still, their weakness can be revealed by evaluating pale and thinned colors of poor saturation or by fast changing of colors in a sample. There can be a tendency also for people with just slightly affected color deficiencies to mistake certain colors under unfavorable conditions (as in dusky weather or fog). This can be unfortunate in situations where fast and precise judgment of colors is essential. It therefore is important that also the slighter degrees of color vision deficiencies are discovered.

## COLOR BLINDNESS AROUND THE WORLD

J. Francois, G. Verriest and collegues at Ghent State University (Francois 1957) found that the percentage of color blind people in populations varied little between the European countries: the frequency in the male population is between 7,2 and 8,8 percent. Non-European people generally show less frequency. Among red-green color defectives, researchers generally agree that the greatest portion, about 50 to 60 percent, is accounted for by green deficiencies (deuteranomals), while red deficiencies (protanomals) account for 12 to 14 percent. Green-blindness (deuteranopia) are generally found in 13 to 18 percent and red-blindness (protanopia) in about 11 percent. The variations weren't great here either.

Red-green blindness is most frequent among white caucasians and less frequent among black people and Australian aborigines (Pickford 1965). Stephen Polyak (cited by Pickford) discusses color vision in evolution. The highest frequency (7 to 8 percent) is found among white people in Europe and in America. In Japan about 5 percent of males are color blind. In India the frequency is 4 to 5 percent and among Native Americans and Australian Aborigines there are about 3 percent. In Polyak's theory. color vision deficiencies are linked with the disadvantage in hunting and collecting food; the lover frequency of color deficiencies in some areas was, in accordance with the theory, a consequence of natural selection in numerous generations.

However, the low prevalence of about 5 percent color blindness in Chinese and Japanese men are revised and doubted by Jennifer Birch in a recent report (Birch 2011). She found that the data about the prevalence rates were generally poorly documented. The reported low prevalence of deficiency in Black Americans was largely derived from small samples. A comprehensive investigation by the US Health Department in 1974 found no significant differences in the prevalence of color defective persons in White and Black Americans.

Terms used for color blindness:

*Color vision defect*
*Color defect*
*Deviating/defective color vision*
*Daltonism*
*Dyschromatopsia*
*Abnormal color vision*
*Color weakness*
*Disturbed color vision*
*Color sense defect*

*Red-green color blindness/ red-green color vision deficiency*
*Blue-yellow color blindness/ Blue-yellow color vision deficiency*

*Total color blindness/ Achromatopsia/ Monochromacy/ Rod monochromacy/ Typical total color blindness.*

# II: WHAT CAUSES COLOR VISION DEFICIENCIES?

# CHAPTER 4: CONGENITAL COLOR VISION DEFICIENCIES

There are two main reasons for congenital color blindness: incorrect pigments in the eye and hereditary disposition.

## INCORRECT PIGMENTS IN THE EYE

Colors are perceived by the brain. The information is taken in by the eyes and the visual pathways, so color vision is an interpretation in the brain of all signals mediated by the visual apparatus. The process starts in the retinal sensory cells —rods and cones (figure 3). The rods, which are the most light sensitive, are in the greatest number. They make it possible to see even in weak illumination. But the cones determine color vision. (It has been calculated that there are 120 millions rods and 6.5 millions cones in the human eye.)

Three kinds of cones contain pigments that are activated by the light. The pigment in each cone is specific and distinct. Signals are sent from the cones through the optic nerve to the brain. Each cone reacts in the same way to light of all wavelengths (the univariance principle), but since not all

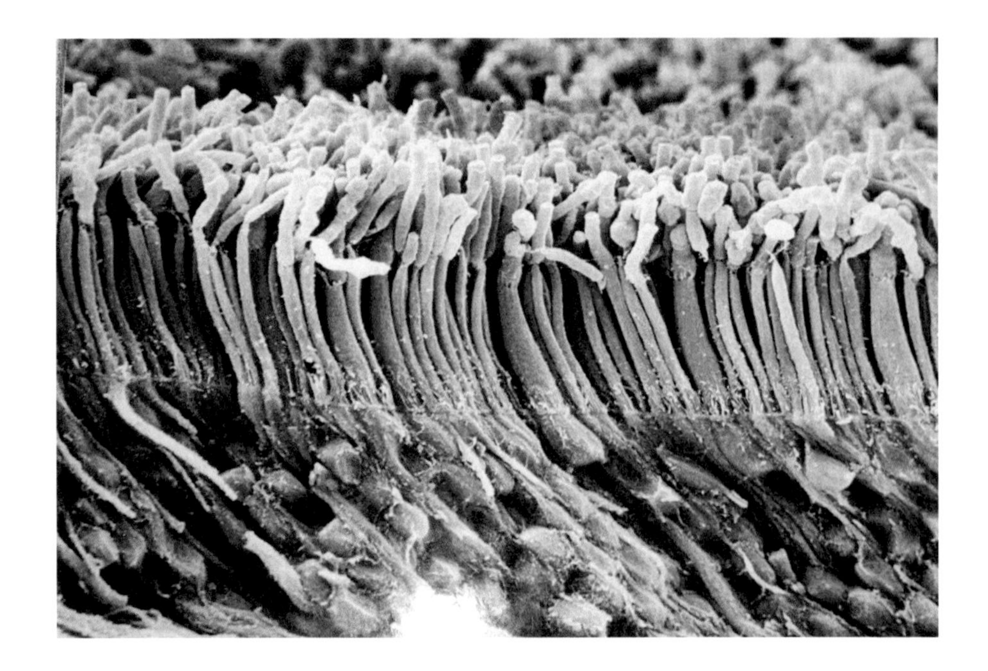

Figure 3. The sense cells in the retina. Electron microscopic picture demonstrating the slim rods and the broader cones (Photo: Martin Davanger).

wavelengths of light fall within the range of the single cone, not all light will be taken up. The role of catching the light of different wavelengths is divided among the different cones. "Red cones" are sensitive to red light and sense light in the long wavelength end of the spectrum. "Green cones" are sensitive to green light and take up light primarily in the middle part of the spectrum. "Blue cones" are sensitive to blue light and sense light in the short wavelength end of the spectrum. There are many more red and relatively few blue cones in the retina. In fact, the ratio of red, green and blue cones is 40:20:1, respectively.[3]

When a person sees a colored object, the three types of cones are activated to a different degree, and each sends a different signal. This is why

3 This ratio comes from Vos and Walraven (Vos 1971); other studies give other estimates of the cone distribution.

we can see innumerable colors with only three types of cones in the retina. Any color in the spectrum can be copied by using a mixture of three other spectral lights. At least three lights from different parts of the spectrum are necessary to achieve a copy of a random spectral color in the normal eye, which is why we call normal color vision *trichromatic.* The color blind need only two different wavelengths to achieve a true copy of a random spectral color; that's why their color vision is said to be *dichromatic.*

> Whether the three cone pigments are complete in number or not, is determining for the color vision.

Scientific development, especially during the last fifty years, has given us more precise knowledge about the color receptors. By studying individuals with deficient color vision, researchers have been able to gain greater knowledge regarding normal color vision as well.

> Precise knowledge of the visual receptors has been obtained by means of specially developed techniques.

Several different theories about what is going on in the retina and how impulses are transmitted have been debated over many years. In 1953, W.A.H. Rushton at the University of Cambridge and R.A. Weale at the University of London were able to demonstrate, independently, through a method called densitometry, that red-green blind individuals possessed only one type of cone pigment when receiving light in the long wavelength part of the spectrum. In this method, the reflection of light from the living eye was measured and compared with the light having been sent into the eye. The lights specified by wavelengths brought forth a characteristic absorption pattern. The phenomenon at play is similar to what we observe when we meet a cat in the darkness and notice the green color of its eyes when the light is shed on it. Something happens to the light when it passes in and out of the cat's eye; the quality of the light has changed. The light is partly absorbed following a certain pattern. Is each cone represented with several types of pigment? Or is there only one type of pigment in the single cone ? This part of the chain of proof was solved in 1964 by W.B. Marks and colleagues, and by P.K. Brown and George Wald. By means of a special method (called micro spectro-photometry) they determined how the different wavelengths of light were absorbed in single cones. They concluded that each single cone contained only one type of pigment. By these methods they measured pigments, not sensations.

Registration of single cone functions is now possible by means of psychophysical methods which make it possible to identify the response of single cone.

In addition to such objective methods, our knowledge has been augmented by fundamental work in the psychophysical and experimental area. Psychophysical means observations based on the patient's sensation. The breakthrough occurred in 1949 by W.S. Stiles in his experiments measuring qualities of light during adaptation to different kinds of background colors (Stiles 1949). Stiles believed that as many as seven cone mechanisms were present in the normal eye. Other works showed only three distinct cone mechanisms. The objective methods are generally preferable, but the psychophysical methods have proven more precise and more practical in measurements of the living eye.

Continued strong light suppresses the activity of the visual cells, making them less sensitive to light stimuli. With special qualities of light, the receptors can be selectively suppressed while others may retain a high degree of sensitivity. In our hospital, the Rikshospital (the National Hospital) I could adapt this principle in developing a clinical method to isolate single color receptors and follow their appearance in the visual field (Hansen 1979). With this method damage of single color mechanisms by disease can be pointed out.

## SUPPRESSING IMPULSES

When the cones are exposed to light, they forward impulses to the brain, but they also generate suppressing impulses which are strong signals. This can be illustrated by the phenomenon called "transient tritanopia." If somebody looks at a surface of uniform yellow color for a while, then a blue point of light on the same surface will appear very clearly. When the yellow light in the background is extinguished, the blue light spot will not appear more distinct, which might be expected, but instead will disappear and remain absent for several seconds before returning. The phenomenon is amazing. It is explained by a blockade of the blue signals in the retina, caused by activities going on in the red- and green-receptors during recovery. When the red- and green receptors are in a phase of regeneration after illumination, they create impulses of suppressing influence on the blue receptors. Transient tritanopia tells us how strong the suppressing impulses can be. It is a normal phenomenon, but is absent if the red- and green-receptors are damaged or missing (as in the case of blue cone monochromacy.)

Figure 4 shows the spectral-sensitivity curves for the three types of cones in the normal eye. Color blindness results when one type of cone is missing. When the red-sensitive cones are not present in the retina, "red blindness" occurs. When green-sensitive cones are missing, we get "green blindness." In both conditions, colors are not distinguished in the long wavelength range (from green up to red), as they have only one active type of cone in that range of the spectrum. All colors in the long wavelength part of the spectrum are seen as variants of yellow, while colors in the short wavelength part are seen as variants of blue. "Blue blindness" arises in the same way if the retina is devoid of blue sensitive cones.

Sometimes, all types of cones are present, but their pigments differ from the normal pattern. For instance, the sensitivity curve of one type

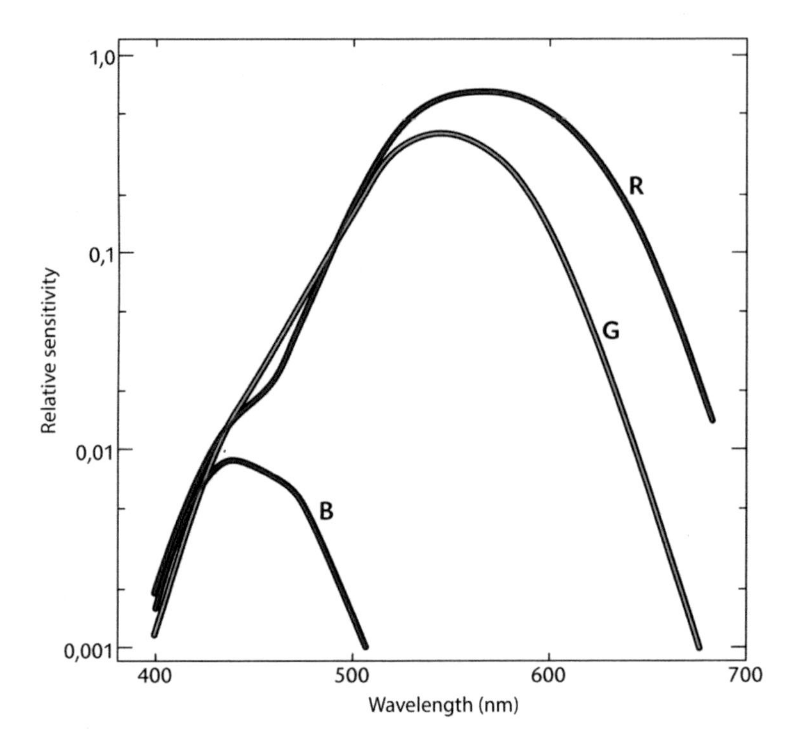


Figure 4. Color sensitivity for three types of cones in the normal eye. B is short-wave sensitive ("blue receptor") cones. G is middle wave-length sensitive ("green receptor") cones. R is long-wavelength sensitive ("red receptor") cones. After Vos and Walraven (Vos 1971).

of cone might be close to the sensitivity curve of another cone. If the sensitivity curve of the red cone is close to the sensitivity curve of the green cone, the differentiation between colors in the long wavelength range will be poor, and we will have the condition called "red weakness" (protanomaly). If the pigment of the green sensitive cone is close to the red cone, we have the condition called "green weakness" (deuteranomaly). In the same way, a deviant curve for the blue sensitive cones can bring about the condition of "blue weakness" (tritanomaly). Nevertheless all of these allow a trichromatic color vision and are therefore named "anomalous trichromats."

## INHERITANCE

Faults in color vision are inborn and remain unchanged throughout life. In certain families they are inherited in a seemingly strange pattern. Typically, they appear in every second generation and almost only in boys. This is because the disposition for color blindness is connected to the sex chromosomes, XX in women and XY in men. In women, the genes for color blindness must be found in both of the two X chromosomes in order for color blindness to be established. Since color blindness is recessive, it will not manifest when suppressed by a normal X chromosome. Women have one X chromosome from each parent. In men it is sufficient to receive one X chromosome for color blindness from the mother in order that color blindness should appear (the Y chromosome, coming from the father, has no dominance). Color blindness in men is thus due to inheritance transmitted from their mother.

Family trees with color blindness started to emerge as early as the 18th century (Berg 1967). Several pedigrees were published during the 19th century. But it took many years before scientists understood how color blindness appeared, disappeared, and then reappeared in successive generations. The heredity of color blindness had great similarity with the transmission of hemophilia (the bleeding disease) which was transmitted from affected grandfathers to their male grandchildren through daughters who were not themselves affected. The Swiss scientist J. F. Horner demonstrated in 1876 that the same rule could be applied to the familiar occurrence of color blindness. The Horner's rule tells that color blindness is transmitted to sons of daughters whose fathers are color blind.

In spite of a large accumulation of data, towards the end of the 19th century scientists had no understanding of the reason why color blindness and color anomalies appeared in families. By about 1911 it was evident that color vision was regulated by genes on the X chromosome and that color vision deficiencies were inherited as a recessive trait.

Gradually, some important publications appeared showing the frequency of various types in the population. In Norway, fundamental research was published by the ophthalmologist Ingolf Schiøtz (1920/22) and by researcher on heredity and forensic medicine, Georg Waaler (1927), see figure 5.

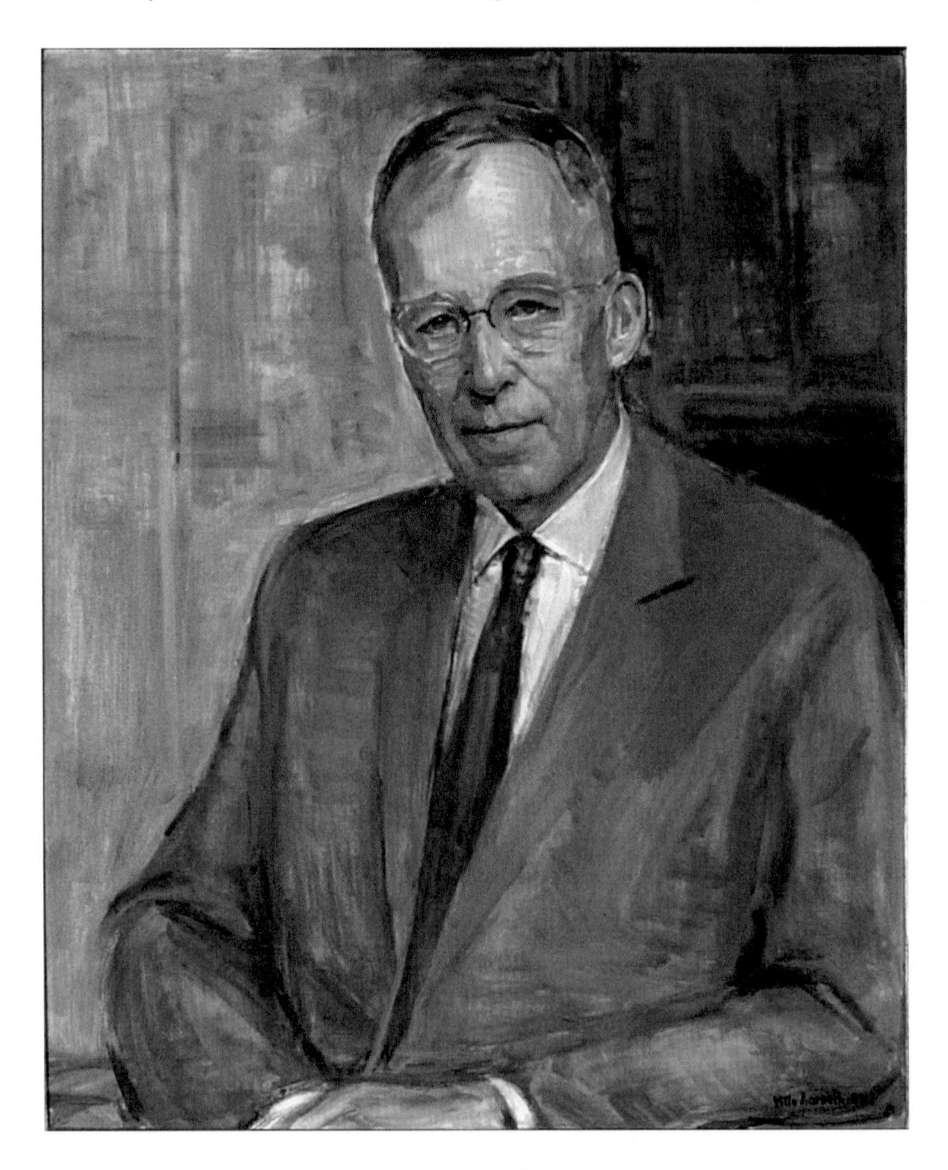

Figure 5. The heredity researcher and expert on forensic medicine George Waaler (1895 - 1983). Painted by Ville Aarseth, the collection of Rikshospitalet, the National Hospital (Photo: Svein Plukkerud).

Schiøtz found a frequency of 10 percent and Waaler 8 percent in men in the population. Both of them confirmed the existence of color blind women, although in a considerable minority. For years before this, since 1878, Anders Daae and others held that "sharper color vision was developed by women because they worked with colored objects over many generations." (Daae 1878).

The incidence of color blindness in men and women is not independent. Statistically one would expect that the incidence in men of 8 percent would imply a frequency of 0.08 x 0.08, or 0.0064 in women. In data from schools of more than 9,000 girls, Waaler in 1927 found 0.44 percent instead of the calculated frequency of 0.64 percent . Waaler was not content with this discrepancy, and he searched for other explanations . He concluded that the gene for green blindness and for red blindness must be located in two different places on the X chromosome, so he launched the new theory, the "two-locus theory." If a woman has the disposition for red blindness in one X chromosome and the disposition for green blindness in her other X chromosome, she will not be color blind because the two genes in different places will overshadow and compensate for each other. Waaler's theory was praised by the well-known New York ophthalmologist Arthur Linksz in his book, *"An Essay on Color Vision"* (Linksz 1964):

*Waaler was the first to give serious thought to the discrepancy between his expected 0.64 per cent for affected females and his actual value - 0.441 per cent. With genius and perseverance he dug into the family pedigrees of afflicted females, studying both their paternal and maternal background, and came up with an explanatory hypothesis which is one of the most brilliant and most remarkable solutions of a biological puzzle.*

We have seen that red-green deficiencies are X-linked recessive inheritance. Daughters of parents who are both color blind, but according to different types, must be normal if the two-locus theory is valid. This proved true in reports from such families.

Waaler's two-locus theory also explains why a woman with normal color vision can have two sons with different types of color deficiency, one with red blindness and the other with green blindness. The X chromosome carrying the gene for the "protan" defect, which one son has received from his mother, is not in the same place as the gene for the "deutan" defect in the mother's second X chromosome, which has been transferred to the other son. The mother thus has one X chromosome with a disposition for red blindness and one X chromosome with a disposition for green blindness. Her XX pattern therefore is consistent with herself having normal color vision.

Variations in the chromosome patterns

*Turner's syndrome* is a curious form of missing menstruation and childlessness. Girls born with this syndrome have an X0 combination of chromosomes (instead of XX). Consequently, the frequency of color deficiency among such girls is at the same level as for boys (i.e. about 8 percent). The occurrence of color blindness is here of special interests, so it is a common routine to send girls with the syndrome for a color-vision examination[4].

In *Klinefelter's syndrome*, afflicted persons have an XXY pattern (i.e. a doubling up of X chromosomes). They may have a male appearance, but weak sex characteristics. The occurrence of color anomalies are rare.

On rare occasions (in 1 of 700 to 1000) a man can have two defective genes in his X chromosome at the same time: a double hemizygote (Kalmus 1965). Color defects in such a case can be difficult to classify. An example of this was a colleague examined by me who had a grave degree of color defect with the characteristics of both protanomaly and deuteranomaly. In 1962, R. W. Pickford reported a double hemizygotic man with combined characteristics of protanomaly and extreme deuteranomaly (Pickford 1962).

Women having genes for color blindness in one X chromosome out of the two X chromosomes generally show normal color vision. Yet in some exceptional cases, women with such (hemizygous) dispositions may manifest different color sensitivities in each eye, being color normal in one eye and color defective in the other eye.

Knowledge of color deficiency can often be used as a "key" in hereditary research. As color deficiency is transferred by special genes in the X chromosome, color blindness can be important as a "marker" in the evaluation of

4 In our department, two women once came in to be evaluated for infertility in the same week, both of whom were color blind.

other hereditary conditions linked to the X chromosomes, like hemophilia which occurs independently of color blindness (as the distance between their genes is great.) In some cases hemophilia and color blindness have been reported to occur in the same family, though this is very seldom even in the same individual. When both occur in one individual, it is referred to as a "crossing over" (Kalmus 1965).

The transference of color blindness as a X-linked recessive inheritance is a characteristic of the red-green deficiency, but is not the case with other types of color deficiencies.

## BLUE-YELLOW COLOR BLINDNESS

Blue-yellow color blindness is most common as an acquired deficiency in connection with other eye diseases. However, it also occurs rarely on its own as a hereditary trait. Known as "Tritan color deficiency," the disorder generally causes less embarrassment than the red-green deficiency. Partly because of this, it is less easily noticed. Blues and yellows are perceived with the greatest difficulty; there is typically confusion with violet, yellow-green, and gray. Other confusions are shown in figure 12.

The precise diagnosis may be uncertain; since other underlying disease conditions can easily be overlooked, determining whether it is acquired or congenital can be difficult. In the Eye Research Laboratories, University of Chicago Alex E. Krill and colleagues, in particular, have been skeptical, doubting the existence of a genuine hereditary blue-yellow deficiency (Krill 1970). This is because the blue-yellow defect commonly occurs as part of a special type of optic-nerve disease, the dominant optic atrophy. However, the damage to the nerve may sometimes be of a small degree and may not significantly influence visual acuity. The condition can therefore be overlooked. All the same, the blue-yellow defect is an acquired one.

Other scientists have documented that genuine hereditary blue-yellow deficiencies are found independently of any other eye diseases. One patient who came to my office had always had problems with blue and green colors.

He had no signs of optic nerve damage or other diseases that could explain his color-vision defect. Gross confusion errors in a tritan pattern were demonstrated and I could confirm blue-yellow color deficiency (figure 6).

In cases of hereditary blue-yellow defects described in the literature, an autosomal dominant heredity has been found: the color vision defect in the affected families occurs in every generation, but with different degree of manifestation. Some members can therefore be affected without having clear symptoms (Kalmus 1965).

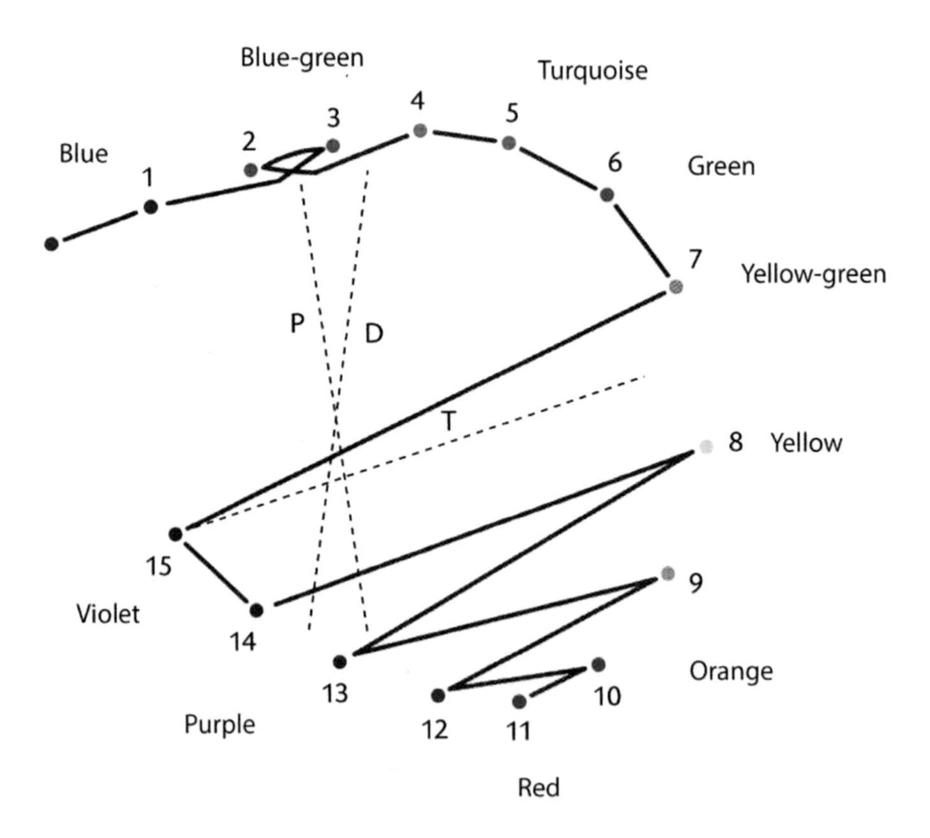


Figure 6. Confusion colors shown with the Farnsworth's D-15 test in a man with congenital blue-yellow color-vision defect. The lines indicate which colors are selected as similar.

Blue-yellow color blind people (tritanopes) have a dichromatic color vision. In other words, all the colors in the spectrum can be made similar to a mixture of two primary colors chosen from the long and short wavelength regions. The neutral point—where the spectrum is colorless and grey—is identified at about 570 nanometers in the yellow-green region. Another neutral point is located in the violet region. The tritan defectives confuse along the axis of violet - grey - yellow green. Parallel confusions are blue and green and also red purple and yellow (figure 12 c). Curiously, blue blindness can be demonstrated in normal eyes in the most central spot (fovea centralis), which is the center for optimal vision.

The diagnosis of blue-yellow deficiency can be made by means of specially designed pseudo-isochromatic charts. The Farnsworth chart II is designed to diagnose red-green as well as blue-yellow deficiency. Such charts are included in the Hardy-Rand-Rittler test, the Stilling test, and the test charts of Hahn. In addition the typical pattern of a tritan defect are revealed by various arrangement tests. Figure 6 shows the confusions for a man with a blue-yellow defect.

Testing blue-yellow defects can also be made with some anomaloscopes by registering matches in the blue-violet and yellow-green region. Also the new lantern test (CAM) constructed by Robert Fletcher is designed to reveal blue-yellow deficiencies.

## TOTAL COLOR BLINDNESS

On rare occasions, color blindness can be complete: the ability to see and differentiate between colors is totally missing. This condition is also called achromatopsia (no color vision) or monochromacy (only one color). It is present from birth and remains unchanged throughout life. The condition, which occurs as often in women as in men, is hereditary and requires a gene from both father and mother. (It is an autosomal recessive trait.) The lack of color vision results when the retina contains only one type of receptor (the rods) to catch all qualities of light. These rods, though, are intact and they function as they do in people with normal color vision.

Typical total color blindness occurs with a frequency of between 1 in 30,000 and 1 in 100,000 in a population. In Norway, for example, 61 people were registered in the Norwegian Registry of Blindness, indicating a prevalence rate of 1 in 70, 000 (The Norwegian Registry of Blindness 1995). The condition can be more concentrated in certain regions: On Fur, a small island in the Limfiord in Denmark, 23 cases of achromatopsia were found in a population of 1600 (Holm 1940). On Pingelap, an isolated island in the Pacific ocean, 57 of about 700 residents were totally color blind, as reported in great detail by the neurologist Oliver Sacks in his book *The Island of the Color Blind.* This condition is called "maskun" by the natives of Pingelap, an estimated one-third of the island's inhabitants carried of the maskun gene (Sacks 1996).

Why these concentrations? Such isolated communities show high rates of intermarriage. Of a Norwegian group of 55 totally color blind people (35 men and 20 women), 31 of them, or 56 percent, knew of other cases in their families, and 13 of them, or 24 percent, had parents who were related in some way, which confirms a link between rates of intermarriage and rates of total color blindness (The Norwegian Registry of Blindness 1995).

The condition is stationary, meaning that no visual deterioration is to be expected. But acchromatopsia is, paradoxically, a condition that is often misdiagnosed by doctors. The visual impairment may be recognized, but then under other diagnoses, like congenital nystagmus, amblyopia, optic nerve atrophy, macular degeneration, ocular albinism, or in some instances cerebral damage.

It is important that a correct diagnosis is made at an early stage. A misdiagnosed child can be regarded as heavily visually-impaired, towards blindness. And when the affected child does not function well in school, he or she can be considered mentally handicapped, with unhappy results. A vivid description is given by the psychologist and researcher Knut Nordby, who was totally color blind (Nordby 1990). His parents were informed that their child would never be able to read or write because of impaired vision and had to go to the school for the blind to learn Braille. The condition was later correctly diagnosed as total color blindness, and Knut was sent to a regular school. Apart from a moderate partial sightlessness, he functioned well in his educational and working life.

Achromatopsia manifests itself at an early age. An aversion to light is the most conspicuous sign, along with an inability to fix the gaze and a characteristic trembling of the eyes (nystagmus). In the areas where the condition is common, it is so noticeable in the newborn that relatives often can confirm that the child has the "heritage" (as it was called by one of the older inhabitants of Fur). But it is not until a later age, when the use of colors and color vision tests can be made that the condition can be confirmed. (Electrophysiological methods can also make an objective diagnosis.)

An inability to discriminate colors is the cardinal symptom and involves all colors in the color circle. Nevertheless, it is possible for the color blind to "recognize" certain colors; for instance, red appears extremely dark, and green appears exceptionally bright. This can confuse people, who cannot believe that the person concerned is totally color blind.

Color discrimination can be partly camouflaged. In school the child learns early to evaluate the colors according to their brightness and by help of their schoolmates to find the right colored pencils for drawing. Quite often at school it is not understood that the fundamental defect is a defect in color vision. Uncertainty and misunderstanding may arise, making the child doubt his or her ability and lose self-confidence. When coloring, the child might use red as a dark color—instead of dark grey. Green, the brightest color in the paintbox, is chosen instead of yellow to illustrate the brightest parts in the drawing (figure 7).

Not unusually the totally color blind may be able to read some of the charts in the Ishihara test, so if the examiner is unfamiliar with color vision testing, he or she might reach the wrong conclusion about whether the person in question is totally color blind. The Ishihara and similar tests are constructed for a normal light distribution, which is different from that for the totally color blind. Their sensation of light distribution is typically scotopic (as in the dark) which can be demonstrated by their performance in arrangement tests like the Farnsworth D-15 test. The diagnosis of total color blindness can also be made by means of the anomaloscope.

Another cardinal symptom is the vibration of the eyes (nystagmus), which in practice is present from birth in all achromats. However, it occurs to varying degrees. As a rule it diminishes with age.

> The most embarrassing symptom is the aversion to light. Besides the lack of color vision there is reduced visual acuity.

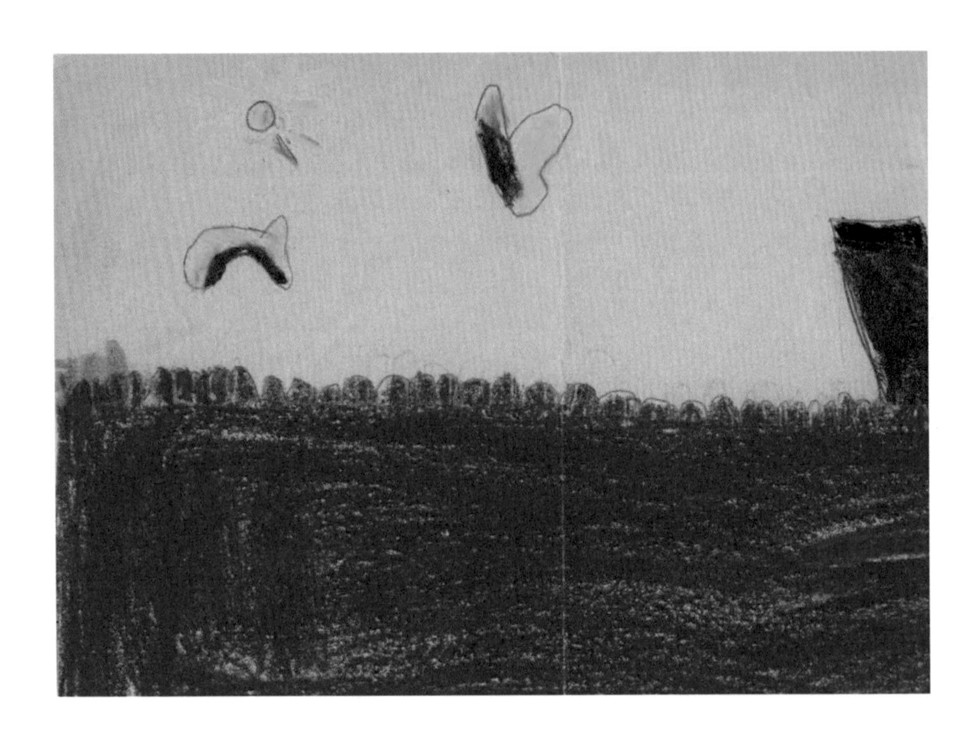

Figure 7. Drawing made by a school child with total color blindness. Green is the brightest color and has been chosen as the color of the sun and the brightest part of the fish.

Aversion to strong light (photophobia) is especially troublesome. The aversion to light is not actually painful, but may manifest itself in involuntary searching for the most shadowy place. At school the child prefers an innermost place in the room. He or she will try to stay away from bright light, especially sunlight, but also clear daylight. Regularly the effect of light is reduced by blinking, squinting or closing one eye. Strong light also annoys: things blended with each other and details disappear. The patients prefer twilight or night lighting, and play in the evening, when they function normally.

Preference for weak lighting is difficult for ordinary people to understand and troublesome for the patient to explain. Many patients would rather ignore the symptoms or explain them away. Sometimes the patient tries to camouflage an urge for dim light. One girl, for example, said she pretended that she was holding books close to her eyes because of her bad vision, while she actually did so to obtain sufficient shadow.

Sports like skiing are problematic, as shadows and contours in the white snow are difficult to distinguish. This is especially difficult under good daylight conditions. White surfaces in general, such as white stairs without dark edges marking the steps, cause problems. All ball games are difficult, because holding on to and following balls in the air depends on good cone vision, which is concentrated in the central part of the retina and is lacking in achromats.

Visual acuity, a measure of visual efficiency, is reduced with achromatopsia, The patients are not in the category of blindness, but are partially sighted, yet the patient still does not meet the requirements for a drivers license. Near vision is relatively better than distance vision. Visual aid can be useful, with some patients preferring an ordinary magnifying glass for close-up work. Consequently they keep away from occupations requiring exposure to a lot of light or demanding especially good vision or work where color vision is important such as architects, interior decorators, florists or TV dealers. Good arrangements, though, allow patients to function well in their working life. Several achromats have obtained higher education and even advanced degrees.

Typical total achromatopsia occurs when there are no functioning cones in the retina. Vision is based on rods only. Rods do not distinguish between light of different wavelengths. The eye is therefore monochromatic, which means that all light appears similar in degree and of the same "color." Thus "monochromacy" is similar to the normal person's experience of seeing colors in very dim light, such as moonlight. Here the relative brightness of the colors is also changed: green is seen as the brightest color while red seems close to complete darkness (known as the Purkinji shift i.e. the change from cone vision to rod vision in very dim light). The receptor cells are differently distributed in the retina, and in the strict central part there are no rod-cells. Ordinarily, in this part of the retina there are only cones to activate the central vision; lack of cones in achromats explains low visual acuity.

In missing cone vision, no suppressing impulses come from the cones when the light is strong. The rods are the most sensitive cells in the eye and enable us to see even in very dim light. Normally a suppression takes place in the rods by a change to cone vision when the illumination increases. However, this suppressing mechanism is missing in the achromats and explains their hypersensitivity to strong light.

Some compensation can be obtained through filters. Red spectacle lenses or slight purple glasses can be useful, as such glasses transmit light only in the long wavelength part of the spectrum where the patient has weak perception. Brown or red-brown tinted contact lenses may dim the light and reduce hypersensitivity to light for some patients.

Paradoxically, achromats can sometimes see fine nuances between samples better than people with normal color vision, even when in other circumstances they make considerable mistakes. One of my patients, a knitter, reported that, when shopping, she was good at picking out pairs of identical nylon stockings belonging together. When knitting, she could differentiate among green threads that appeared identical to sales staff. On the other hand, she used red instead of blue yarn in her knitting; yellow napkins appeared white; she thought a red-headed woman was a brunette; and she could hardly see writing in green or green lines on blankets.

A network has been established for collecting and sharing information about this rare eye condition, and it has its own journal; *The Achromatopsia*

*Network Newsletter.* (The contact person is Frances Futterman, P.O. Box 214, Berkeley, California, USA, 94701-0214.)

## SPECIAL TYPES OF ACHROMATOPSIA

There are also incomplete forms in addition to the typical total color blindness. In *Blue cone monochromacy,* blue cones are present together with the rods in their retina. These people are visually impaired. The condition is the best-known type of incomplete achromatopsia.

*Cone monochromacy* is an exceptionally rare variant. Only a few cases have been described. Despite the presence of functioning cones in the retina, these persons are totally color blind. They see the world in shades of white and black. They are not light-sensitive, and their visual acuity is normal.

*Progressive cone dystrophy* refers to a progressive deterioration of color vision ending with total color blindness. There is a congenital disposition. In Hansen-Larsen-Berg's syndrome progressive cone dystrophy occurs together with liver degeneration and endocrine disorder (Hansen 1976).

# CHAPTER 5: ACQUIRED COLOR VISION DEFECTS

Loose estimates suggest that as many as five percent of the population may have acquired color vision defects; this holds especially for the blue-yellow type. This is not inconceivable in view of the many diseases and injuries that can affect the visual system, many of which go unnoticed. They must be traced by more fine-grained methods.

Color vision is easily influenced by changes in the visual system. An old rule, Köllner's rule, says that diseases in the outer retinal layer generally cause disturbances in blue-yellow color vision while diseases affecting the inner retinal layer usually cause red-green disturbances. Köllner's rule can be verified in many cases, but does not so far have general validity. Color-vision defects can occur as side effects from drugs and intoxicants. Side effects from medication can often be detected earlier by color vision testing than by conventional methods. Medication can influence the visual apparatus at different levels. Acquired color vision defects can be side effects of general disease or caused by eye disease, or damage to the eye, the optic nerve, or the visual tract. A group of special character deals with damage occurring in the higher visual centers.

Acquired defects may resemble congenital ones, but are essentially different from congenital defects caused by hereditary pigment deviations in the receptor cells. They are not, like congenital defects, stationary and unchangeable. The beginning can be insidious. They are often related to one side and are less specific. Numerous disease conditions in the eye and in the visual apparatus also affect color vision. I have included in this review only some examples; references to the many other diseases involving color vision defects can be found in the specialized literature.

Normal color vision changes with age. Color weakness is almost a normal physiological phenomenon at a higher age, marked by a reduced ability to discriminate subtle color differences. This is clearly demonstrated with the Farnsworth - Munsell 100 Hue test, where a higher error score is found for older patients. For example, Guy Verriest found that color vision gradually deteriorates with age, especially for the blue sensitivity and a weakening along the blue-yellow axis (Verriest 1971). Cloudiness in the anterior part of the eye, as with cataract, also leads to changes in color perception. With cataract the changes occur so slowly as to be unnoticed by the person concerned. However, when the cloudy lens is removed by an operation, there can be a striking change. One of my patients told me that the blue and violet colors looked entirely clear after an operation, while the same colors looked weak and diffuse before the operation. Another patient expressed the change in this way: things he thought were gray (tools etc.) turned out to be blue. What he thought were dull green turned out to be clear blue.

The above-mentioned cases are examples from modern cataract operations when an artificial lens is installed with properties close to the natural lens, as opposed to operations undertaken in earlier times, when the cloudy lens was removed without installation of a new lens (this is still the procedure in many developing countries due to lack of resources, and the resulting condition, called aphakia (without lens) results in a more drastic change in color perception).

Lawrence Spitalny and his co-researchers (Spitalny 1969) described how an artist experienced the change between his normal eye and his operated (aphakic) eye. If he painted a motif first with his normal eye and then, after regarding the picture with his aphakic eye, picked out the colors and copied the same motif, there was a striking difference: the blue sky was reproduced now in intense deep blue. Orange-red was fuchsia. Yellow green grass was painted sharper green by changing the color hue towards blue-green. There was a loss of the warmer nuances of color. This double set of paintings illustrated the change of color hue perception in the aphakic eye. The change of color in the aphakic eye could be compensated by a slightly brown-colored contact lens.

The example with cataract illustrates the special type of influence on color perception caused by clouding of the ocular media (an absorption system). The same effect on color vision can result from cloudiness of the cornea due to different causes. The absorption system involves changes occurring in front of the receptor cells unlike changes occurring in the receptor cells themselves or the nerve system (a reduction system).

Acquired color vision defects are classified into different types without being identical with the congenital defects. According to the well-known color-vision researcher Guy Verriest (Verriest 1963), the acquired defects can be classified into three groups:

* *Type I* has some resemblance with the congenital protan deficiency. There is a gradual deterioration of the red-green discrimination and at the same time a reduction of visual acuity. The brightness of the long wavelength part of the spectrum is reduced and at an advanced stage is close to total color blindness.
* *Type II* comprises red-green defects of another type with spectral brightness distribution as in a normal person. This type can also deteriorate. It resembles congenital deutan deficiency.
* *Type III* is characterized by a lack of sensitivity to blue and has resemblance with the congenital blue-yellow deficiency (tritan defect). The sensitivity to blue is especially the case for many disease conditions in the eye, making type III the most frequent of the acquired color vision defects.

It is important that color-vision disturbances are diagnosed as they may be an early symptom of diseases, especially those caused by intoxication and the adverse influence of medicines. In some cases color vision defects can be the key to understanding vague disease conditions. Color vision examinations are also a useful aid in following up similar conditions.

## INTOXICATIONS

Adverse effect of medicine

*Digitalis* is a frequently used medicine in heart disease. It can cause such side effects as yellow-colored vision, blurred vision, and flickering spots in the visual field. In one case of color vision defect type I from using digitalis, there was increased sensitivity to blue and a grave loss of sensitivity to colors at the red end of the spectrum. (Gibson 1965). Examination in the anomaloscope confirmed a marked red weakness, which, however, disappeared gradually. The 100 Hue test demonstrated a great loss of ability to discriminate colors in several parts of the color circle. The symptoms were temporary and disappeared when digitalis was no longer taken.

Digitalis may sometimes induce chromatopsias (green vision or yellow vision) when taken over time. The yellowish paintings of van Gogh could possibly be explained by his use of digitalis, among other remedies (Marmor 2009).

> Vision damage can easily occur because of contact with several toxic ingredients in addition to medicines having adverse effects.

*Optic nerve intoxication* can be the cause of color blindness type II. A good survey of color vision defects caused by medicines is given by Wolfgang Jaeger and Hermann Krastel (Jaeger 1987 ). Color vision examination is very important in detecting the early stages of optic nerve intoxication and for follow-ups.

Vision can be damaged by over-use of tobacco. This type of visual damage (tobacco amblyopia) used to be common, but is seldom seen today. In this regard color vision is an important indicator for following the disease condition. Here the 100 Hue test is especially useful.

Etambutol and Neambutol, commonly used as remedies for tuberculosis, can cause a red-green defect of type II. A further deterioration of color vision can also occur in patients with congenital color vision deficiency, as I found in one of my patients after his prolonged use of Etambutol.

Jaeger and Krastel found an increase of width of the receptive fields in the retina due to optic nerve damage caused by pharmacotherapy. Patients could only read the color charts at a shorter distance; the authors therefore proposed "reading at a short distance" as a new test for optic nerve damage. Monoamine-oxidase-inhibitor, the medicine formerly used to treat high blood pressure and depression, caused a red-green defect of type II. The patients could not see the different colors of traffic signals. Their color vision was restored when the treatment was stopped.

Kinin and Kinidin, a remedy for malaria, can lead to toxic damage of the optic nerve; so can Optochin and Eucupin. All of them can result in blindness. In general toxic nerve damage is a recurring cause of type II red-green defect.

Chloroquine and the Chloroquine derivatives are all toxic and can cause both blue-yellow defects and red-green defects. Chloroquine was originally a remedy for combating malaria and proved to be effective in treating rheumatism. In the beginning , in the 60ths and 70ths, the medicine could be freely bought. However, after repeated use, some patients sustained serious damage to their retina. In my hospital, for example, one patient reported having a curious color vision defect: a red thread seemed to change between sections of red and black. Also a blue thread changed between sections of light blue and dull blue. She tended to confuse dark gray and red and blue and yellow. She could not make out writing in blue pen on bluish paper. Closer analysis of her receptor pattern revealed a *selective* influence on the receptor cells. The rod vision was relatively stable. The red and green sensitive cones in the early stage were clearly malfunctioning. Typically among our patients was a loss of color vision in a narrow field just outside the center of sharp vision (4-6 degrees from central fixation), while the central field itself functioned well. A lack of response from the red and green sensitive cones in a confined area outside the center of the visual field was thus confirmed, while the blue cone response was little affected.

## DISEASES IN THE EYE AND THE VISUAL PATHWAYS

Color-vision defects caused by disease can be mild or severe. The mild defects, also the most commonly occurring, are often overlooked. The type of color defect can often be an indication of the localization of the disease process. The eye's blue mechanism is especially vulnerable by many acquired diseases. For instance, a blue-yellow defect by glaucoma can indicate an effect on the outer layers in the retina, and a red-green defect by macular degeneration in young people can indicate damage chiefly to the nerve cell layer.

*Age related macular degeneration (AMD)*, often called "calcification," is among the most common causes of visual deficiency in elderly patients. Blue-yellow deficiency and also red-green deficiency can be found, but the blue-yellow deficiency is predominant. In his book "Recent advances in the study of the acquired deficiencies of colour vision," Guy Verriest found deficiency of blue sensitivity (type III defect) in most of his patients with a moderate accompanying red-green defect (Verriest 1974). The sensitivity for red was less than for green. Verriest stated that color vision disturbance is an early manifestation of age related macular defect, because even in cases with good visual acuity, a severe color vision disturbance is possible. A weakened blue-yellow discrimination was also found to be out to 20 degrees peripherally.

*Retinitis pigmentosa* most typically leads to a blue-yellow defect (type III). One of my patients, a nurse, could not see the markings made with yellow in the daily journal report. When the changes are merely concentrated in the periphery, visual acuity and the central color vision is most often normal. However, when the central vision is affected, a red-green deficiency (type I) can also occur. Reduced sensitivity for blue can be demonstrated by the measurement of selective color receptor sensitivity (Hansen 1979).

*Stargardt's disease (juvenile macular degeneration)* is a retinal degeneration occurring in young children. Here the typical finding is a red-green color defect as distinct from the blue-yellow defect found in AMD (age related macular degeneration), which is typical in the elderly. Stargardt's disease is the classical example of a type I red-green defect. The typical color confusion pattern can easily be shown with the Farnsworth D-15 test. In the anomaloscope, a reduced sensitivity for long wavelength (red) light is registered, which later can expand towards green. Further development of the disease can occur through protanopia (red blindness) and eventually total color blindness. The retinal degeneration in its classical form is limited to the central area.

*Stengel's disease* (the Batten-Mayo/ Spielmeyer-Stock's disease) has a more serious prognosis [5]. It hits children at an early age (about 4 to 5 years). The color vision defect is a typical red-green defect (type I), which at advanced stage can make the patient blind, especially for long wavelength light. For example, one of our patients could not see at all when examined during a strong yellow background light (from a Sodium (Na) lamp.) On the contrary, her vision in white light and in short wavelength (blue) light was fairly good.

*Diabetes* brings about a disturbance of color vision of minor degree. With the 100 Hue test, which is the most sensitive test, the error score for all ages is higher in diabetics than in the population in general. This also applies to patients without visible changes in their eyes, but is even higher when retinal changes are present (Pokorny 1979). Yet good color vision can be a common finding even in spite of insufficient regulation. Treatment of retinal changes by using lasers is frequently carried out and in many patients to an extensive degree. Even some patients who have had laser therapy to hinder the progression of the disease give near normal error score on the arrangement tests, but the majority show a drastic increase in the number of errors (Kurtenbach 2001). The many point defects in the retina caused by laser treatment are generally unnoticed by the patients, but they can still be traced by registration of the more delicate color discrimination.

*Glaucoma* brings about color vision defects of type III blue-yellow defect, usually with a good response of the red and green stimuli. However, red-green defects have also been reported. The sensitivity of all receptor cells are relatively weakened, but especially the "blue mechanism" may be damaged. An early sign of damage from glaucoma is shown by a weakening of the sensitivity to blue lights in the visual field. It is now established as a method

---

5 Most correctly the name Stengel, as the first author to describe the disease (Stengel 1826), should be linked to the disease.

in the newer perimeters where the sensitivity to blue stimulating lights are registered during adaptation to a homogenous yellow background light. The degree of the color vision defect is related to the visual field defect. It can be shown in a simple way by the Farnsworth's D-15 test.

For *damage to the optic nerve (optic nerve atrophy)*, color-vision examination is an important method to differentiate among types of disease. The mild, dominantly inherited form is characteristically a blue-yellow defect (type III). It is very similar to the congenital type of blue-yellow defect (tritanopia), a recognized condition but occurring in extremely few people. The great similarity has made some researchers believe that there is no congenital type of blue-yellow defect. This is supported by the fact that many patients with dominantly inherited optic atrophy have little weakening of their visual acuity and may pass as normally seeing people (Krill 1970). The other type of optic atrophy, the *Leber optic atrophy*, is a disease with a far more serious reduction of visual function. Here the typical finding is a red-green deficiency (type II).

Another type is optic nerve affection in connection with general disease that has consequences for color vision. Recently a man aged 56, a train engineer, was referred to me by the railway doctor because of difficulties in distinguishing shades of color. He had been afflicted by multiple sclerosis and had partly reduced visual acuity. In contrast to earlier examinations he could no longer read the color plates. His settings in the anomaloscope were in the normal range but widely spread. There was no increased color contrast sensitivity and normal brightness values. He exhibited a typical red-green color defect of acquired type II.

> Eye diseases often have an influence on color vision because they often damage visual receptor cells or nerve connections which are important to color vision.

Color-vision defects from damaging events are not infrequent and can, like congenital defects, have highly different degrees of defect. However, they are experienced in a different way. First, the patients themselves often realize that change has occurred with their color vision. (in people with congenital defects, color vision remains what it always has been). Another characteristic by the acquired type is that the color vision disturbance generally is not stationary or unchangeable. On the contrary, it can progress from mild to more pronounced disturbance. Or it can be temporary. Acquired defects are expressions of the basic affliction (for instance intoxication or as a side effect of a medicine) and are most often in both eyes. Selected injury or disease usually results in a color vision defect in one eye only.

## DAMAGE OF CEREBRAL CENTERS

> The brain undertakes certain operations for construction of color on the basis of information from the outside.

The experience of color is initiated when the signals from the eye reach the brain. How does it happen? Where in the brain does it take place?

For a long time scientists viewed color as the wavelength composition of the light being reflected from an object. However, strictly speaking, radiated light has no color (as stated by Newton). Yet light rays have the ability to initiate in the brain the sensation of one color or another. The code here can be the dominance of the wavelengths reflecting from the object. All that is demanded from the brain is decoding the message (Zeki 1999).

But if the brain's experience of color is exclusively dependent on wavelengths, then the color of objects would continuously change as light changes. Then the objects would no longer even be recognized as a certain color. But we experience the colors of objects as constant. How can this be? And where in the brain is the correction taking place?

The brain undertakes an operation. It registers the relation between the light of a given wavelength that is reflected from an object and the light of the same wavelength reflected from the surroundings. *Colors constancy* is the phenomenon of ignoring changes and maintaining the colors. By drawing a comparison between the wavelength compositions, the brain makes a construction of the color and presents it with an interpretation. Seeing colors is then a mental process taking place all the time.

Several areas in the brain are involved. In his book *Inner Vision,* Semir Zeki reports recent findings that make it possible to explain the process. Area VI (the visual cortex in the posterior part of the brain) gives the initial information. Here wavelength-sensitive cells receive impulses from the receptor cells in the retina. They respond only to light of a given wavelength. If this center was the only center for color vision, our surroundings would appear highly confusing with continuously changing colors.

Poisoning from carbon monoxide (from car exhaust or gas) can cause a kind of blindness, but patients who survive it can still see and report different colors in spite of their blindness. V. S. Ramachandran reports on a tragic accident where a woman almost died after washing her hair using warm water from a gas burner with defective ventilation (Ramachandran 2005). Miraculously, she was saved, but completely blind when she awakened from a coma. After a few days, though, she could recognize colors, but her perception of colors was altered. She could not keep focused on a constant color. The failing here was lack of adaptation of the color impulses (the wavelength-determined signals) in another cerebral area, which could be called the color vision center. This patient could only describe the correct color of a surface when the surface was reflecting the same color in abundance. Thus, color constancy was missing, but not wavelength perception.

The visual center in the brain is localized in the cerebral cortex in area VI (Figure 8). During the color process, area VI is also the active area in a normal person. However, there is another area which is even more active, the V4-complex (V4 and V4@) on the underside of the brain. Semir Zeki proved that this area is the seat of the comparative mechanism giving rise to color constancy (Zeki 1973) . Partial damage of V4 causes a condition where the person in question is unable to see the colors as constant characters (which means being no longer independent of changing illumination). Total damage of the V4 area, which occasionally is seen, causes a total loss of color vision, called *cerebral achromatopsia.*

Oliver Sacks has described this condition in *The Case of the Colorblind Painter.* After a traffic accident, a patient suddenly experienced total color blindness. His brown dog was grayish. The tomato juice was dark. Not only had colors vanished; what he saw, was "dirty" and unappetizing. Skin colors looked like the colors of a rat. His own paintings seemed repulsive. Tests revealed that he was able to distinguish different wavelengths. However, he could not make the jump from there to the interpretation of the wavelengths as colors. He was unable to generate the cerebral and mental imagination of colors (Sacks 1995).

This was due to a selective damage in the brain affecting only the V4 area. It was a permanent state in this patient. Thereby, a special center for color vision in the brain was demonstrated. This had been presumed earlier, but had never been proved. It had even been denied by some authorities that such a center existed. In the 1920s, the prominent neurologist Gordon Holmes investigated 200 cases of vision complaints after bullet wounds in the visual cortex and did not find a single case of cerebral color blindness. He declared that an isolated cerebral achromatopsia could not occur. This contributed to stopping all clinical interest on this question.

But after the detection of Semir Zeki in 1973, several reports of cerebral damage involving the V4 center with color vision defects were published. Damasio and coworkers (Damasio 1980) in Iowa explained why Holmes did not find any cases of color defects in his material: his patients had defects in the upper part of the visual cortex (in V1), while the damaged center that causes achromatopsia is on the underside of the brain (in V4).

Acquired cerebral dyschromatopsia (partial color blindness) was reported by Glenn Green and Simmons Lessel in 1977. Five of their patients had lesions in the posterior part of the visual cortex. This indicated that affection of the lower part of the visual brain could be responsible for the acquired cerebral color blindness, as well as another curious phenomenon, the loss of ability to recognize faces (prosopagnosia). This was one of the earliest case reports pointing to the existence of a cerebral center for color vision (Green 1977).

Color vision loss can also occur as a temporal phenomenon by cerebral damage (also by embolism). Immediately after a hip operation, one of my patients, a 76-year-old woman, saw everything in gray. After one week, she began seeing colors again, but the colors of cloths and furniture were confused and "wrong." When I saw her again two months later, she had regained normal color vision.

After a dramatic preeclampsia going over to ecclampsia, another patient of mine was brought to the hospital in a coma. When she awoke, she was blind for several days, but thereafter her vision gradually returned. But it was confused, and she saw things in the surroundings dislocated as in Picasso's cubist paintings. The colors then gradually returned, but were fluttering and questionable. The visual disturbance was temporary.

A. Ogata and coworkers in Japan have described a 75-year-old woman who complained of disturbed color vision and difficulties in recognizing forms and faces following a sudden blindness that lasted an hour (Ogata 2005). She had an infarct in the cerebral area near to the visual center (gyrus fusiformis), which was in addition to a bigger earlier infarct in the visual cortex on the other side of the brain. Her color vision defect was also temporary.

Jack Moreland and coworkers (Moreland 1995) tell of a man with a complete loss of color vision after brain infection (encephalitis) caused unconsciousness. His color vision partly returned in the course of 20 months, but he reported that the colors were no longer as he remembered. His ability to discriminate and name colors was damaged. There was imprecise and unstable perception of colors by changes of illumination. Cerebral damage was ascertained to be around the V4 visual center. The receptor cells in the retina proved to be normal upon examination.

A curious defect reported by A.R. Damasio and H. Damasio called "color anomia" can occur by damage of the visual cortex in the anterior part of the left gyrus lingualis (Area V3 close to the visual center in V4). (Damasio 1992). These patients see colors as normal. But they have lost the ability to name the colors correctly. If a green or a yellow color is shown to them, they may identify them as blue or red. But when asked to carry out matching of colors, they perform it correctly. The defect is thus connected to the naming of the colors rather than the perception of them.

Josef Zihl reports on disturbed color vision as a result of cerebral damage in the posterior and the middle part of the brain (occipitotemporal) (Zihl 2000). It can be on one side and may then be expressed as a disturbance in the upper half of the opposite visual field. The patients remark that the colors are "very pale" or "like an old film." It is a selective disturbance— a loss only of the color vision. Double-sided damage of the same areas can cause a weakness of color perception in the entire visual field, but except for extreme cases, not a complete loss of color vision (cerebral achromatopsia). Zihl supposes it is possible to improve color vision in such cases by special training (based on documentation from two of his patients).

Color vision defects due to cerebral damage are different from congenital defects in several ways:

* The defects do not follow a particular pattern, but are random.
* The patients do not see the test charts based on confusion patterns in the color vision tests (the "camouflage" test charts) which are easily readable for other color deficient persons.
* Visual field defects are often present. With one sided lesions, the color vision loss may be restricted to one side (for instance only in the right visual field).

Because of proximity to other cerebral centers, color vision defects can occur together with other disturbances of the sensory apparatus. Injury to certain cerebral areas may give rise to specific confusions.

The retina is closely connected to the primary visual cortex in V1 which has also been called "the cortical retina" (figure 8). Next to this is the visual association region (prestriate cortex), which is in several sections. Damage of V2 can lead to so-called "mind blindness," a condition where the individual can see, but is not able to understand what he or she is seeing, which is distinct from damage to the V1 causing a real visual loss (Derefeldt 1993). A certain specializing of the visual cortex is going on all the time in the way that color, form and movement take place in separate processes.

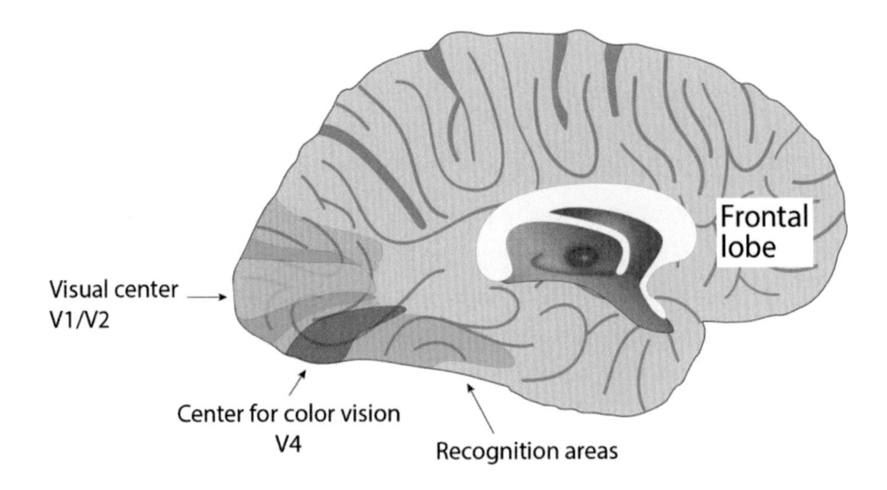


Figure 8. The visual centers in the brain relevant for color vision. The left half of the brain seen from the inner side. Modified after (Zeki 1999).

# III: HOW DO WE TEST FOR COLOR VISION?

# CHAPTER 6: TESTS FOR EXAMINING COLOR VISION

Careful testing is required when there are doubts about a person's color vision. A simple examination consisting of choosing certain objects and asking for their color is insufficient, as the person in question may be good at recognizing the colors of familiar objects in the surroundings.

*A man had been sent to me for a color vision examination as he had applied for a dispensation to work in the security service in the railway sector. As he doubted the result of my examination and my diagnosis of a color vision defect, he therefore applied for a new examination and came this time together with two trade union colleagues. They stated that the applicant, after being confronted with several colors, had always named the colors correctly and therefore could not be color blind. However, some simple color tests revealed a grave confusion of colors, and now everybody was convinced of the diagnosis.*

Several common tests are suitable to disclose certain weaknesses characteristic for different types of color deficiency.

## SYSTEMATIZING COLORS

To understanding the problem with color-vision defects, it may be useful to look at the systems used for arranging colors. In the swarm of colors, some combinations of colors seem to harmonize better than others.

Leonardo da Vinci favored red and green over other pairs of colors. The contrasts with these colors gave the best color combinations. Also Goethe pointed out a kind of relationship between colors like the pairs red/green and yellow/blue. The colors here were suppressing each other and at the same time emphasizing each other. This two-sided influence was among others cited in support of Hering's opponent color theory (1886), which was a counterpart to the prevailing theory of Young-Helmholtz. There are an almost endless number of colors in our surroundings. There have been attempts to find ways in arranging colors for better surveillance of all the changing nuances.

There are three main characteristics for determining colors:

* *Hue or chromaticity* determines the shade of color or color nuance.
* *Saturation* or *chroma* indicates the strength of hue or richness of color.
* *Brightness,* indicating the clarity, the degree of whiteness/darkness or luminosity.

Most commonly, the order of the colors are presented around a circle according to the hue. The criterion for the location of the colors is varied. It can be done schematically, as in the Hering's color circle where the main colors red - yellow - green - and blue are separated by the same distance in the circle and are filled in with the intermediate colors. Another way is to make each step in the color circle like the smallest possible difference in hue that can be recognized by normal observers. With colors of similar saturation and brightness, the sample of colors can be arranged in a circle. This is what we find in Munsell's object color circle. Here each step is determined, as mentioned above, by the physiological principle of the least possible difference in hue. This color circle is also called "the physiological color circle ." In the Munsell system, 100 defined colors surround the center; in this arrangement, it is possible to distinguish 100 different color hues, although 100 is taken as a somewhat schematic number. The Farnsworth-Munsell 100 hue test, based on the Muncell's color circle, contains 85 chips. This practical test can very well illustrate where in the color system the weakness of color perception is found (figure 9).

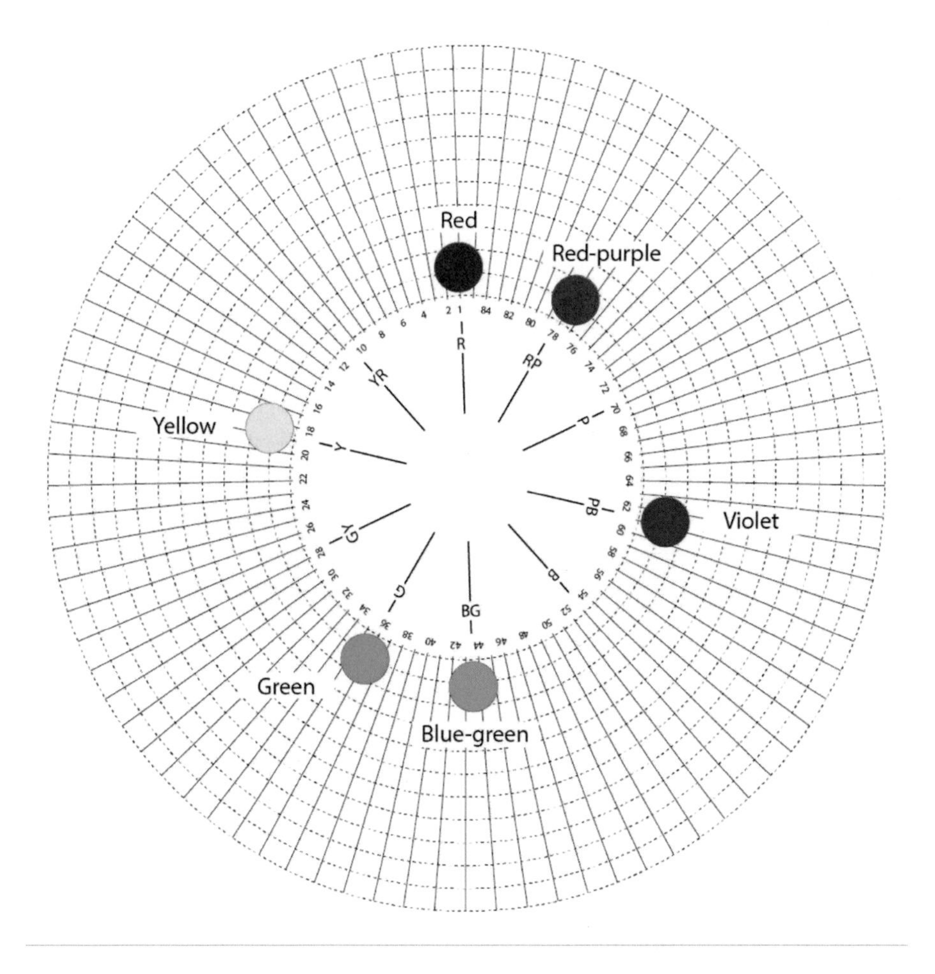


Figure 9. The color steps in the Farnsworth-Munsell 100 Hue test as expressed by "the physiological color circle." Each step represents the smallest noticeable hue difference which can normally be recognized. The complementary colors are found diametrically opposite to each other. Notice that red is opposite to blue-green and green is opposite to red-purple.

## FARNSWORTH-MUNSELL 100 HUE TEST

This is a test of how well one can differentiate between subtle color nuances, i.e. seeing the differences between hues close to each other on the color circle. The examinee is asked to arrange the chips in accordance with similarity of colors within a limited part of the color circle. The colored chips are presented in mixed order in wooden cases, each of which contains a quarter of the full range color circle.

Contrary to many color vision tests where correct score can be normally expected, this is a very sensitive test where under normal circumstances also some errors are expected to be made. The test provides a quantification of the quality of the color discrimination. However, of even greater interest, the test reveals where in the circle most errors are found. Protans (P and PA)—those who experience one main type of red-green defect— make the most mistakes in the region of purple to purple-blue colors and in the yellow-green region. Deutans (D and DA)—who experience the other main type— have the highest error score in the blue to blue-purple color region and in the yellow to yellow-red region. These regions are then quite different from the regions with *poorest* saturation, i. e. in the blue-green and red areas for the protans and in the green and red-purple areas for the deutans. On the contrary, here people with color-vision deficiency have no or very few errors on the 100 Hue test, despite their color vision being distinctively poor in those areas. Accordingly, here we have uncovered a paradox. It has been formulated as *Pitt's law:* "Differential wave length discrimination in the color defective is best where color saturation is poorest," as reported by Arthur Linksz (1964).

This ability to discriminate color differences can be extremely well developed and may even surpass the normal sighted person's ability. Patients with red-green color defect have at various times told about their special ability in seeing tints of colors better than others. In a hospital where I once worked, the technical head, who was "green blind" (deuteranope), corrected a painted color made by another member of the staff for matching a green surface. Everyone thought the color was correct, but the chief was unsatisfied and mixed the paints to obtain another tint of green as a better match, which was then also accepted by the others.

## DESATURATION

A main point regarding color deficiency is color desaturation, which takes place when some colors are seen as very pale or even colorless. When those with color-vision deficiencies say that colors are desaturated, the normally sighted see the same colors as strong, with good saturation. This is obviously a shortage in the measurement of color. The degree of desaturation may be varied. For mild types of color-vision deficiency, with only a small degree of desaturation present, they may not noticeably mistake color estimation. In the most pronounced forms (as in dichromatic color vision) these colors are not only weak, but are totally missing. It means that instead of seeing a distinct color as is seen by the normally sighted, they are here seeing only a grey or white area. This deficiency is usually limited to certain areas in the color circle or only specified wavelengths in a spectrum. These limited areas are found for the protanope (the red blind) in the blue-green region and for the deuteranope (the green blind) in the pure green region. Just here the regions are colorless. For the less-pronounced types of color defects the corresponding areas are colored, but the colors appear distinctively weak (colorless). This is in contrast to the neighbor colors which may have relatively good saturation.

Arthur Linksz, in his book "An Essay on Color Vision," states how the spectral colors are perceived. For the normal eye, the weakest saturation is found in the yellow-green region (about 565 nanometers). For the partially red blind, and the partially green blind, the color saturation in the same region is also weak, but the region of maximum poor saturation is found at about 490 nm and at about 500 nm for the protanomal and the deuteranomal, respectively (Linksz 1964). So there are especially weak regions of saturation in the blue-green (490 nm) and the green (500 nm) regions, where the colors are experienced as being very pale and nearly colorless. The narrow areas here are distinctly different for the red defectives (PA) and the green defectives (DA) (figure 10). The red blind (P) and the green blind (D) are seeing the same areas respectively as completely colorless (gray).

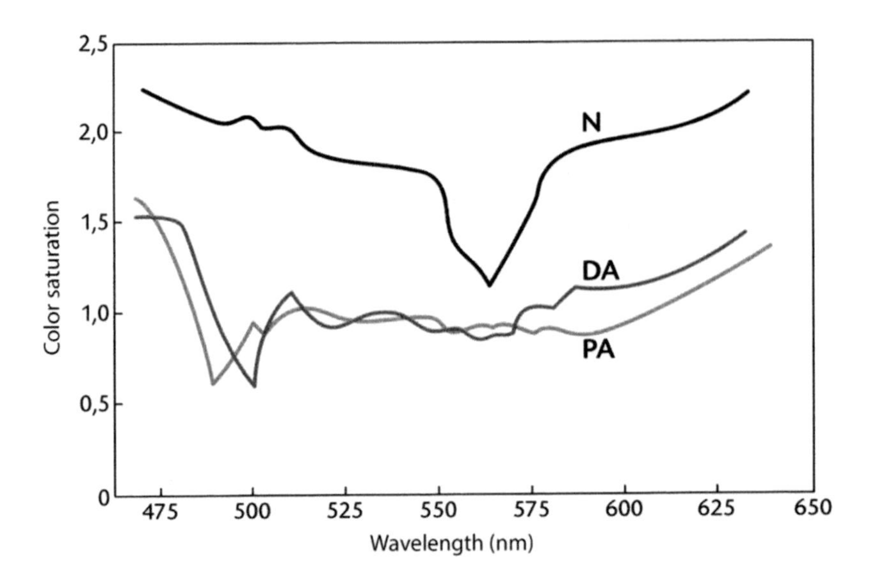


Figure 10. The saturation of colors in different parts of the spectrum in the normal (N), the deuteranomal (DA) and the protanomal (PA). Maximum desaturation is in the blue-green region (at about 490 nm for the PA) and the green region (at about 500 nm for the DA). The people with more pronounced color-vision deficiency, the protanope (P) and deuteranope (D) are seeing the spectrum here colorless (gray) at the corresponding wavelengths. Yellow-green (about 560 nm) is the color of poorest saturation for the normally sighted. Modified after Chapanis (Chapanis 1944).

## THE HARDY-RAND-RITTLER TEST

A more exact diagnosis of color-vision defects, pointing out the weak areas in the color circle, is revealing. Some of the tests just aim to present figures of dominating wavelengths, which are especially critical for people with color-vision deficiency. This is best illustrated by the charts in the Hardy-Rand-Rittler test. Adjusted for the two types of red-green deficiencies, the figures are made in two variants of green: one of blue-green hue and one of pure green hue. The red blind and the red weak persons (the protans) can hardly see the figures presented in blue-green color, while the green blind and the green weak persons (the deutans) can hardly see the green figures. These various tints of green may seem very similar to people with normal color vision, but to the red-green defective they are markedly different. They may be able to see one of the hue qualities, while the other quality may be totally absent.

There are also other deficiencies than those connected to the two green values. For better understanding we need to go back to the color circle (the physiological color circle), where red is opposite , or complementary, to blue green and red-purple to green. Where one of the colors is weakened, the complementary color is also weakened. When there is a failure to see a blue-green color, there is likewise a failure in seeing the red color (for the protan). When there is a weak perception of green, there is also a failure in seeing red-purple (for the deutan). The color blinds are in this way both red blind and green blind. Therefore some of the charts in the Hardy-Rand-Rittler test have figures of red and red-purple values. There are likewise charts for testing blue-yellow color vision with figures partly of violet and yellow-green tints and partly of blue and yellow tints.

The HRR color vision test (developed by LeGrand Hardy, Gertrud Rand and Catherine Rittler) is different from other pseudo-isochromatic tests, in that it is a qualitative test deciding the *type* of color deficiency (figure 11) and at the same time a quantitative test deciding the *degree* of color defect (whether it is of mild, average or pronounced degree).

## CONFUSED COLORS

The pattern of confusion is characteristic for each type of color defect:

* The protane defective (P and PA) confuses colors along the main axis *blue-green - gray - and red*
* The deutane defective (D and DA) confuses colors along the main axis *green - gray - and red- purple*
* The tritane defective (T and TA) confuses colors along the main axis *violet - gray - and yellow-green*

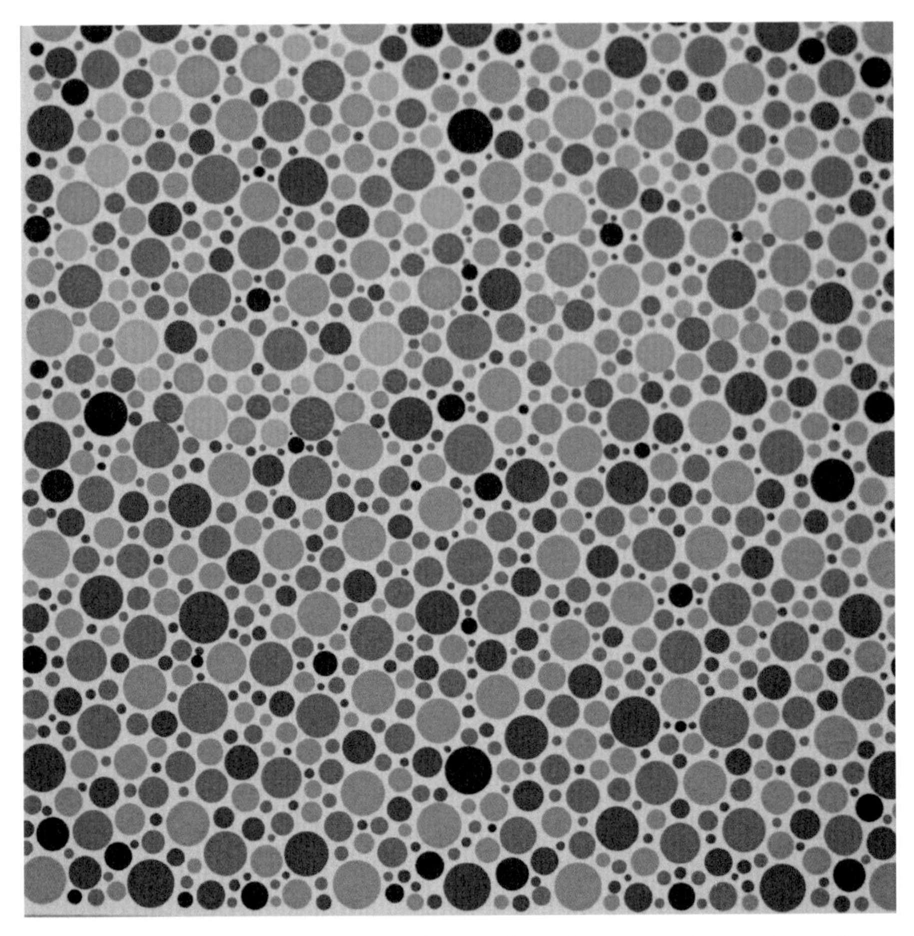

Figure 11. Chart from the Hardy-Rand-Rittler test with two tints of green. The green deficients (the deutans) may be able to see the blue-green figure, but not the green figure. The red deficients (the protans) may be able to see the green figure, but not the blue-green figure.

The confusion of color hues is not accidental, but follows a certain pattern. The confusion colors are different for the red blind (the protane) and the green blind (the deutane).

When the colors mentioned here are so mutually weak as to be confused, it is to be expected that the combined colors with these components can also be confused. It is also the case for the protane defective where blue for red-purple and also green for red-orange can be mistaken. The deutane defective can easily confuse blue-green with purple and likewise red with brown, olive and yellow-green.

The current confusion-mistakes made by the color defective is well presented in Farnsworth's iso-color diagram (Farnsworth 1951). A modified form of which is shown in figure 12.

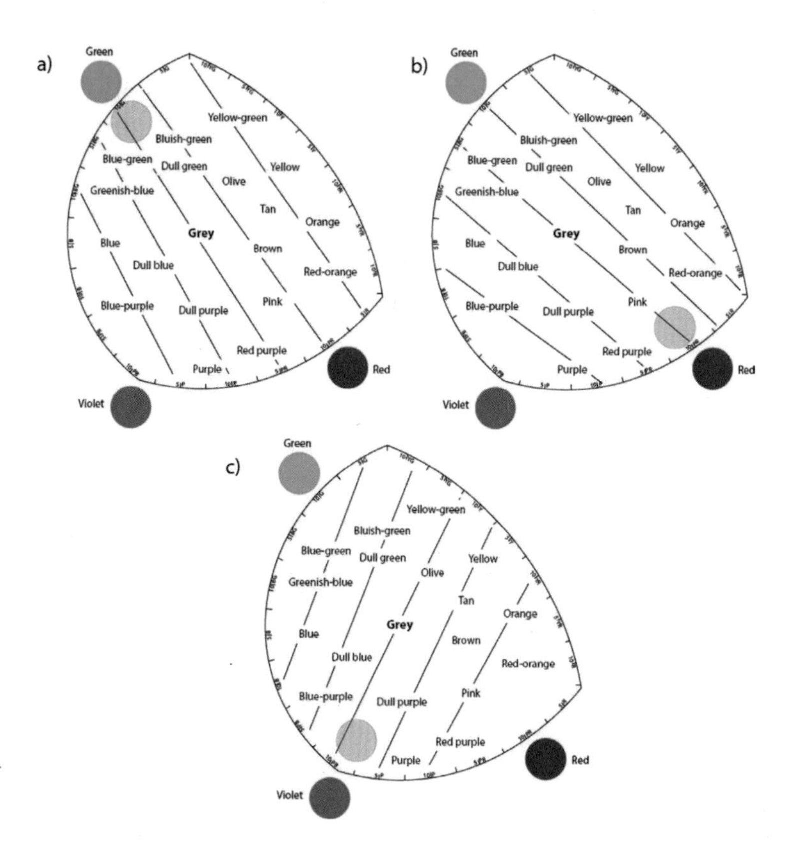


Figure 12. Characteristic confusion colors for each type of color defect. The lines indicate the colors that are most easily confused. a) for the deutane (the green blind), b) for the protane (the red blind) and c) for the tritane (the blue blind); modified after the Farnsworth's iso-color diagram (Farnsworth 1951).

## FARNSWORTH'S D-15-TEST

In 1947 the American naval doctor D. Farnsworth introduced his Dichotomous Test for Color Blindness, Panel D-15. The test displays how the color blinds confuse dissimilar colors. This test is different from the 100 Hue Test, which is for discriminating near-related color tints. The Farnswort's D-15-test is designed to reveal gross confusions of colors, and it reveals only those with a more serious color vision defect. The examinee is asked to arrange a small selection of colored chips (15) in such a way that the chips with greatest similarity will be next to each other (figure 13). Depending on which colors are mistaken or mixed together, a pattern will appear. There are characteristic patterns for each type of color defect. They are hardly accidental—rather the order is logical and "correct" to the person with a color-vision deficiency. Typically the test is carried out in the same way or nearly the same way each time. It allows us to see how the mistakes are distributed and along which axes they occur, making it possible to make diagnoses concerning the type of color-vision defect. The pattern of mistakes is different for protan, deutan, and tritan defectives (see figure 12).

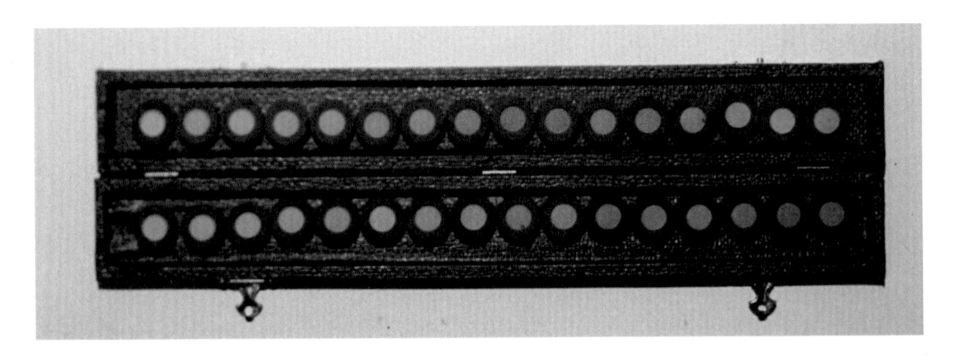

Figure 13. Farnsworth's Dichotomous Test for Color Blindness. In the upper panel, performed in correct order. In the bottom panel, performed by a "green blind" (deuteranope).

## CONTRAST COLORS

Evaluation of color is to a great degree influenced by the surroundings, and when several colors are seen together, their shades of color tint may be changed. This is well known by artists and is utilized to achieve painting effects. There is an inherent tendency to see the alternate color next to the main color. The colors emphasize each other. This is also built into the way the eye is organized and works.

## INCREASED CONTRAST SENSITIVITY

Quite often, color blind people have a vivid sensation of increased color contrast with colors of high chromaticity. This is a characteristic of the moderately color blind (the anomal trichromats). Protanomalous and the deuteranomalous may see the neighbor neutral color (gray) next to a clear red or green area as a vivid contrast color in green or red, respectively. And a tritan person may see a gray area next to a clear blue as yellow. A color stimulus thus brings out the opposite, or the complementary color.

The phenomenon, which is called *simultaneous contrast*, is especially strong for the anomalous trichromats. Here they demonstrate an increased contrast sensitivity that immediately could be regarded as an expression of a good color perception (figure 14). Investigations, however, show that instead of good color sensitivity, it is indicative of a *deficient* color perception. The increased color sensitivity which is manifested, is thus apparent, and the phenomenon therefore is called *falsely increased contrast sensitivity.*

While it is the weak color hues that elicit contrast colors in the normally sighted person, the strong color hues bring about the vivid "counter colors" in the color defective.

Another phenomenon is the *after contrast.* When colors are rapidly changing, the color-defective person (the anomalous trichromat) may point out a wrong color for a neutral (white or yellow) light after having first seen a clear red or green light. This counter color may be seen as a strong and vivid color, sometimes quite as strong as the main color.

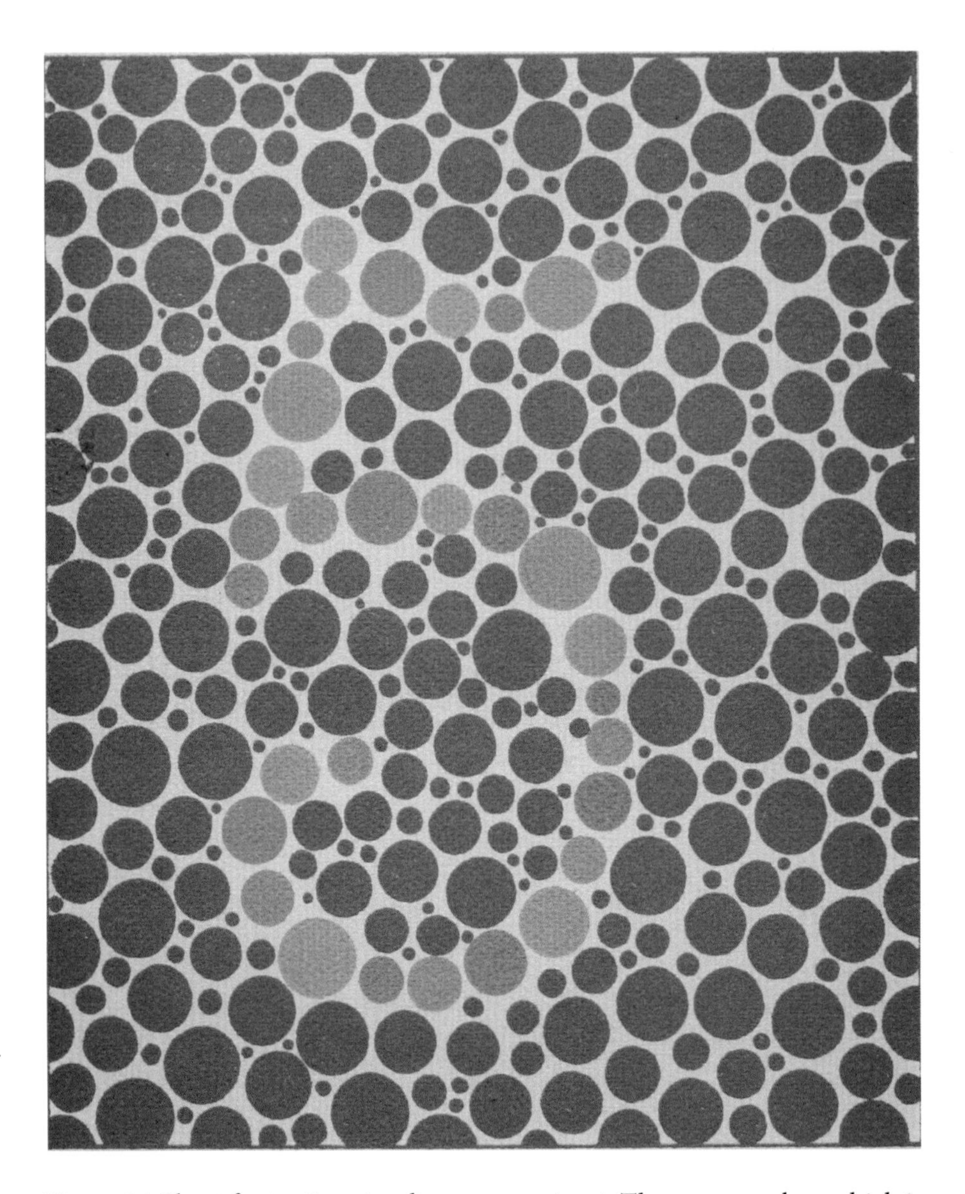

Figure 14 Chart for testing simultaneous contrast. The grey number, which is seen against a clear red background, can be seen by many people with color-vision deficiency as green. Reproduced from the Stilling test (21st edition).

The color-weak people (the protanomalous and the deuteranomalous) in that respect demonstrate an impairment which can be very disturbing in the evaluation of colors: They see the typical contrast colors both shortly after having seen strong colors and when seeing strong colors next to grey or white. This apparent increased contrast sensitivity is in fact an indication of a weakened color vision. The phenomenon of falsely increased contrast sensitivity does not occur in the more pronounced types of color deficiency (in the protanope and the deuteranope) nor in people with normal color vision. Falsely increased contrast sensitivity can be particularly dangerous in persons who are not aware of their color deficiency. This may therefore be an important factor to evaluate in the security services for railway, sea, and aviation. Falsely increased contrast sensitivity can also explain why some people with color-vision deficiency are unable to maintain a constant impression of color even on large areas when the main color and the contrast color change to dominate the picture.

## TISSUE-PAPER CONTRAST TESTS

Contrast sensitivity is caused by strong impulses, which normally make themselves felt in different ways that can be registered. The contrast phenomenon is noticed, as mentioned above, when seeing different areas next to each other (simultaneous contrast) or seeing rapidly changing color lights (after contrast). Specific tests, the tissue paper contrast tests, are designed in such a way that they are seen when the color perception is good (as is the case for people with normal color vision) but fail when the color perception is weak.

In figure 15, we see two contrast charts. When covered by a partly translucent tissue paper, the contours are blurred and the color field is weakened, but can still be faintly seen through the paper. The central, neutral gray figures show through the paper, but are even weaker and in some instances not visible. Nevertheless, this pale and blurred background color makes us see the gray figures because it brings out a counter color (the complementary color to the colored surface). This is the case for the normally sighted, but when the color vision is impaired, as is the case for the anomalous trichromats, the background color will appear too weak for producing a counter color, and no figures will be seen.

The tissue-paper contrast test is selective in the sense that the background colors determine how the different types of color defectives lose recognition of the figures (Hansen 1976). The protanomalous (the red defectives) mainly miss the charts with red or blue-green background colors, while the deuteranomalous (the green defectives) primarily miss the charts with red-purple and green background colors.

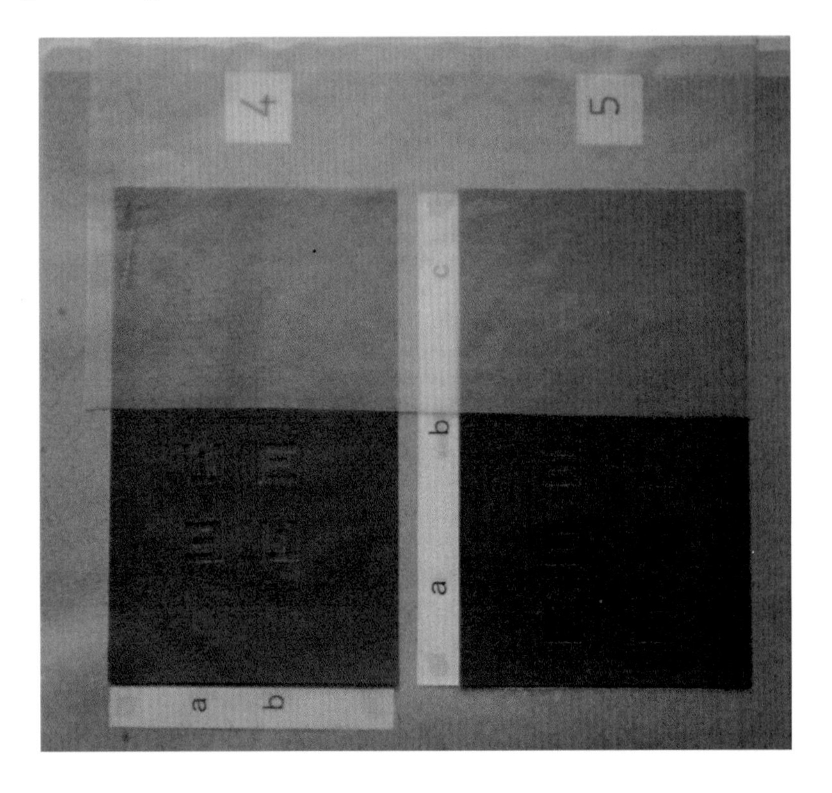


Figure 15 Tissue-paper contrast tests. By covering the charts with tissue paper, the E-figures become invisible when the examinee has impaired contrast sensitivity. Having good color perception is a characteristic for the normally sighted, and the E-figures can still be seen through the tissue paper because of the induction of a counter color within the neutral (gray) areas. The figures on the left chart (red-purple) are not seen by the deuteranomalous and the figures on the right chart (red) not by the protanomalous.

## PSEUDO-ISOCHROMATIC CHARTS

This type of chart is designed with numbers and letters made up with colors that are often confused by the person with a color-vision deficiency. As we have seen, the first test charts of this type were introduced by Stilling in 1878. The test charts were called "pseudo-isochromatic" (meaning apparently of the same color). This was a completely new principle that simplified the procedure and made testing easier to decide whether people had normal or defective color vision. One did not need to ask the examinee which colors he was seeing, only which forms he could recognize.

The Stilling test was met with much skepticism when it was introduced in Germany, probably because of the over-diagnosing of color blindness. At that time, the real prevalence of the mild degrees of color vision deficiencies had not been discovered.

Later, the Stilling test appeared in many editions. It increasingly gained currency and was considered as a reliable test. It also included some charts for testing blue-yellow defects. New editions were also sent out with additional charts and under new names (Hertel-Stilling and, later, Velhagen).

Among the many different types of pseudo-isochromatic tests, the most extensively used is the Japanese Ishihara *test.* In many quarters, examination of color vision is nearly synonymous with the Ishihara test. In Scandinavia, the Boström-Kugelberg test was also considered reliable. All three tests (Stilling, Ishihara, and B-K) were accepted for approval for testing applicants for the merchant navy. For testing young children there are special tests (figure 17).

A series of pseudo-isochromatic charts designed by Hahn in South Korea has more recently come out. While earlier test charts were constructed with empirically chosen confusion colors, the colors of the test figures in Hahn's test are determined by the knowledge of the critical confusion colors for people with color-vision deficiency (figure 16). These figures have great similarity with the Ishihara test charts, and are at about the same level of sensitivity.

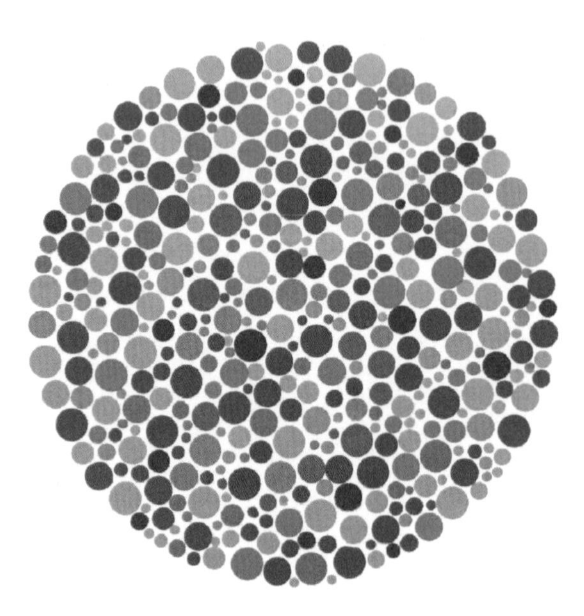

Figure 16 a). A chart reproduced from the Hahn's series of pseudo-isochromatic charts. The number that is visible for the normally sighted, is constructed to be invisible for people with color-vision deficiency.

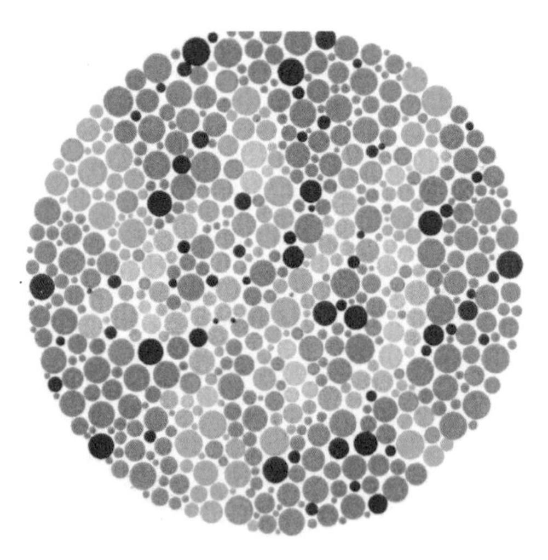

Figure 16 b). "Hidden digit" chart from the ishihara test. Observers with normal color vision are distracted from seeing the faintly grayish figure (45) which is usually seen clearly by people with color deficiency.

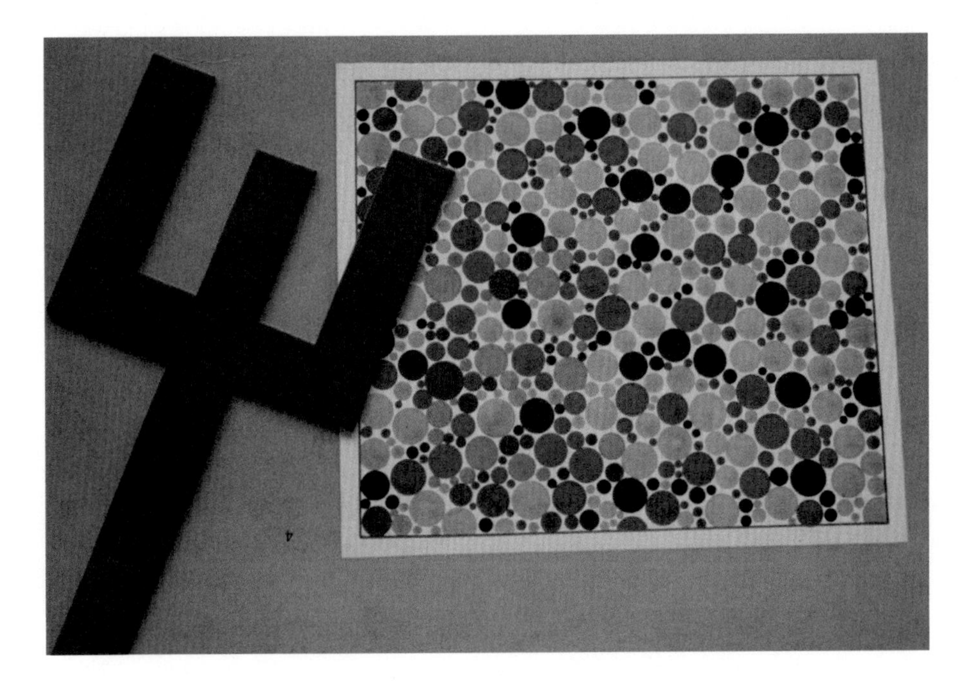

Figure 17. Reproduction from Velhagen's pseudo-isochromatic charts for children with E-figures, which can be identified by means of an attached hook. (Velhagen 1980).

The pseudo-isochromatic charts are supposed to be easily and precisely read by all normally sighted, while the people with color-vision deficiency are expected not to be able to read the figures. But it is necessary to use a series of charts to get a reliable impression of the examinee's color vision. Some normally sighted people can read the figures hesitantly or with errors. That is because they may be more or less familiar with the forms used. On the other hand, certain exceptional people with color-vision deficiency may be able to read nearly a whole series of charts correctly, and they will not be diagnosed with color-vision deficiencies. However, most people with color-vision deficiency, including those with a mild affliction, do commit some mistakes, or they may see the figures hesitantly. In that way they may give away their color deficiency. A gray area exists where mistakes and uncertainty can be shown among bad readers, among color deficient, as well as among normal individuals.

## HIDDEN DIGITS (CAMOUFLAGE TESTS)

Besides the regular pseudo-isochromatic charts, there are charts with an *opposite* effect: they cause people with normal color vision to make errors by missing digits which at the same time may be visible to people with color vision deficiency, who are not so easily distracted by the colorful lines in irregular patterns. The purpose of the charts is to demonstrate color deficiency in a more positive way; that is, making the figures visible to those with a red-green deficiency, but not to normal observers, for whom they are "hidden digits," and are therefore often called "camouflage test charts." (figure 16 b).

## TESTING CONDITIONS

Accurate testing of color vision is dependent on proper conditions. The examiner should be familiar with the tests. The tests, which are constructed to be seen under certain light, should be shown under correct illumination. Ordinary daylight is usually well suited for examination, though with no direct sunshine. Artificial illumination can be used if it is comparable with daylight. Daylight source C (specified by the International Commission of Illumination) is the defined standard for color vision examination. Spectacles with tinted glasses should not be used and certainly not colored filters. (Filters deceive but are not a real compensation for color-vision deficiency).

The tests should be done in full, as no single test gives a complete picture of a color defect. A battery of tests should be used, administered by those with proper training.

> *A worst case example is a story told from a military camp. A sergeant testing the recruits for the officer candidate school presented the charts from the Ishihara test by giving one single chart for each recruit. One wrong answer meant "not accepted for the officer candidate school."*

Insufficient or shallow examination of color vision can cause unfair harm, especially when someone might have to give up a professional career later on in life because of an incorrect test early in life. A wrong acceptance sometimes occurs. More seldom is the opposite consequence. I once met a man who had wanted to start a career as a naval officer and was informed that he had a deficient color vision and could not be accepted for service on deck. He changed to another working career. Then, in old age he applied for exemption to sail his own boat for leisure. A correctly performed examination proved that his color vision was normal!

Although the functional handicap of color-vision deficiency in itself is minimal, it is of importance to know about any possible color vision defect. Usually the first examination of color vision takes place at school. A more complete examination for those falling out should be undertaken and together with their parents be followed up with adequate information.

## ARRANGEMENT TESTS

With these tests, the examinee himself carries out the arrangement of the colors to the best of his judgment, or he/she makes a choice of preferred colors. The tests give a valuable hint of the nature of the color disturbance by showing the characteristic patterns for the various types of color defect. They are thus useful as diagnostic tests. Among the arrangement tests are the Farnsworth-Munsell 100 Hue test and the Farnsworth Panel D-15 test (described earlier).

As a rule those with a mild degree of color deficiency may have a normal performance on the simple arrangement tests ((the Farnsworth Panel D-15 test and the Hahn's D-15 test). There are still several types of arrangement tests, of which some have varying degrees of color saturation aimed at revealing the milder degrees of color-vision deficiency. Some of these are:

* Lanthony's saturated and unsaturated test, which includes chips in gray tints.
* Sahlgren's test, with some chips in gray tints, is especially fitted to test acquired color vision loss.
* Hahn's saturated and desaturated test, which is constructed in accordance with the Farnsworth's Panel D-15 test._

The City University Colour Vision Test (constructed by Robert Fletcher in 1972 and based on Farnsworth's Panel D-15 and Daae's test) displays the typical confusion colors for different types of color deficiencies presented on 10 charts (Fletcher 1972). Each of the 10 charts contains a central reference color and four surrounding colors. The patient is asked to point out which one of the surrounding colors has the greatest similarity to the central color ("forced choice"). There are four possible choices: normal - tritan - protan - deutan (figure 18). The City University test reveals the color defects of medium and severe degrees, and its efficiency is at about the same level as the Farnsworth's D-15 test (Oliphant 1998).

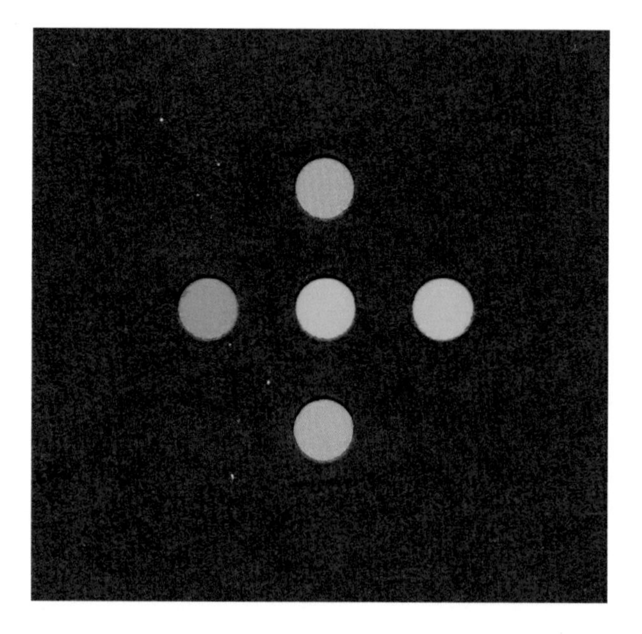

Figure 18. Chart from the City University Colour Vision Test. The examinee is asked to point out the color being most similar to the central test color. Correct choice is the color to the right. If he points out the uppermost color (red), it indicates a protan defect. If the lower color (red-purple) is chosen, it indicates a deutan defect, and the color to the left (green) a tritan defect.

## ANOMALOSCOPE

In the anomaloscope one can find out which colors are deteriorated and how much.

By mixing monochromatic red light with monochromatic green light, Lord Rayleigh found that the resulting color was indistinguishable from a monochromatic yellow light. The relative relation of red/green quantity was variable, but within small limits for the great majority of people. Relative quantity was described by an equation, now known as *Rayleigh's equation.*

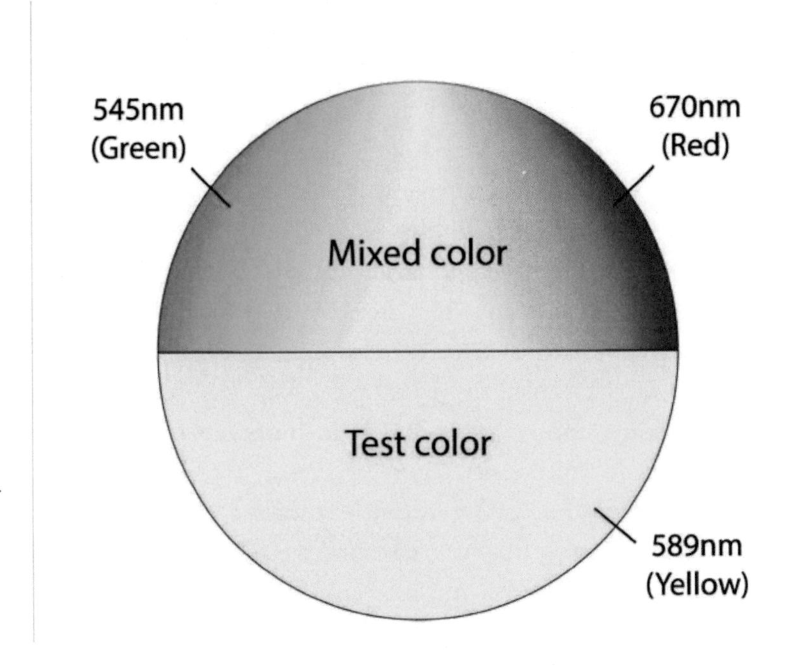


Figure 19. The color fields of the anomaloscope. In the upper field the patient adjusts the mixture of red and green until there is a match with the yellow lower field. In the same way the brightness of the lower field can be adjusted.

In 1907, W.A. Nagel constructed an apparatus, the anomaloscope, which easily can be used to set the Rayleigh equation. The apparatus is very precise, using spectral lights which are monochromatic. The mixing colors are red (wavelength 670 nm) and yellow-green (wavelength 545 nm) in one section, which is matched with a constant yellow field (wavelength 589 nm) (figure 19). Both people with normal and defective color vision are able to do adjustments to obtain a perfect match of the two fields. The normally sighted people adjust the mixture of red and green lights with settings at nearly the same level for matching the yellow field.

The people with color-vision deficiency (anomalous trichromats) stand out by using red and green in quite different proportions. The red defective people mix in more red, while the green defective persons mix more green in order to get a match with the yellow field. Here the fluctuations are considerably larger. The deviations can be expressed as anomalous quotients (AQ) indicating the amount of green in relation to the amount of red light. Unsteady color vision is revealed by a great scattering of the settings. The seriously color blind (the dichromats) accept the spectral colors red and green in all proportions as equivalent to yellow. The diagnosis can be made by the relative brightness of the colored lights. Red is seen as a very dark color by the red blind (the protanope) who therefore have to adjust the yellow field to low brightness value for a match. The green blind (the deuteranope) obtain a match with the yellow field at normal brightness value.

In addition to the Nagel anomaloscope, which uses spectral lights, the Tomey anomaloscope, using diodes, has been introduced. Others have constructed anomaloscope by use of interference filters. With the Nagel II anomaloscope, other parts of the spectrum can be used for examining blue-yellow deficiencies. A disadvantage here was the difference of color saturation. This has been rectified in the Moreland anomaloscope and in the Tomey anomaloscope.

## LANTERN TESTS

The simplest and earliest test is the lantern test introduced in England about 1853 and in France about 1858. (See the earlier description in Chapter 2.).

With a lantern test, one creates an illusion of the real lights from lanterns and lighthouses used at sea. It is a direct test of the ability to recognize the main colors red and green in addition to testing the ability to distinguish these colors from neutral lights (white or yellow). Different kinds of lantern tests are in use. They either can show the lights one by one, and the examinee is asked to indicate the displayed color,or they can present two colors together for testing whether the patient can differentiate the colors correctly. It is likewise a test of the *simultaneous contrast,* which can cause trouble, especially among the partly color blind (anomalous trichromats), who have a tendency to perceive a counter color in the field next to a field of strong red or green.

The lantern tests are easy to understand, and they imitate practical working conditions. Many have confidence in the lantern tests for deciding whether the applicants do or do not fulfill basic vision requirements to ensure safety. Many authorities find it convenient to rely on only one single test, which is why they prefer the lantern test. However, it would not be right to trust only one such test. Some normally sighted people can occasionally make a mistake, and some with serious color defect can happen to perform the test well. Moreover, the tests are not standardized, so the outcome of the examination is dependent on how they are administered. Generally, lantern tests are being used to confirm what is already known from other tests. They should be *supplementary* tests, not primary tests.

Hjalmar Schiøtz in Norway was one of the first to construct a color torch with changeable filters showing the actual colors. The advantage with this was the flashing light that made it easy to test the falsely increased *after-contrast,* which is usually found in anomalous trichromats. The Edridge-Green's lantern, the Giles-Archer lantern and the Holmes-Wright's color lantern have been among the commonly used lantern tests, but are no longer commercially available. A new lantern test has recently been constructed by Robert Fletcher at London City University (Fletcher 2005). In the U.S. , the Farnsworth's lantern test has been widely used and is now replaced by a more simple Farnsworth flashlight lantern which is suitable to test the simultaneous contrast sensitivity. A more elaborate lantern test is the PAPI system (see chapter 10) used in aviation testing procedures and also the CAD (Color Assessment and Diagnosis) test.

# IV: RAMIFICATIONS OF COLOR BLINDNESS

# CHAPTER 7: OTHER DISTURBANCES OF COLOR VISION

Sometimes color vision can play tricks on us. As mentioned earlier, judging colors is influenced by neighboring colors, which can make a color change its character. Such changes are well documented. But under special conditions, such distortions can seem like an occurrence of color blindness.

1) Most people know how our perception of color vanishes in twilight or moonlight. Colors turn into shades of gray, but they also change their brightness. Green becomes the brightest color, with the tree leaves shining in light colors; red appears dark, nearly black. That is because the eye's cones don't function in dim light. A shift to rod vision, known as the *Purkinji shift*, takes place. The rods have a huge potential in dim light. A consequence of the change to rod vision in such a weak illumination is that there also is a displacement of the eye's maximum sensitivity. Contrary to what is expected, sensitivity and contrast become centered outside the point of fixation (maximum sensitivity by night vision is 12 to 15 degrees peripherally). It is difficult to undertake complicated activities at night; therefore it is necessary to learn to see differently in the dark. For example during the Second World War, Norwegian soldiers in England during training were ordered to play football in the dark so as to be capable of night service.

The estimation of colors is weakened when viewed against a dark area, even when the landscape is otherwise clear. Red objects are particularly hard to assess. This was demonstrated by a tragic hunting accident in the mountains some years ago when a man was shot by a hunting colleague as he came in from a dark part of the wood wearing a red cap for a warning. His silhouette was seen indistinctly and was taken for a roe deer. Here the red color served more as camouflage than warning color.

2) At the other extreme, extraordinary strong light can also be a disturbance of color vision. A young man, after intense sunbathing, experienced that the color hues were changed and appeared strange, even though he had kept his eyes shut. Yellow spots appeared pink, then desaturated; blue-green appeared blue. Confusion of colors was noticeable especially in the blue-green region. I saw him at our clinic nine days after exposure, where I found a deterioration especially of the blue sensitive mechanism; it persisted after seven months (Hansen 1980). Color deficiency can also be artificially induced in experiments by strong light of certain wavelengths, which was first shown by W.S. Stiles (Stiles 1949).

## VULNERABLE RETINAL RECEPTORS

The blue sensitive cones, in particular, are vulnerable to external influence. In extraordinarily strong lighting, for instance—such as the intense blue light used by dentists during the hardening process of dental material— damage of visual acuity and color vision can occur. Dentists have to use spectacles shutting off the short wavelength light. Sometimes the intense blue light can cause permanent damage of the blue receptors, which was demonstrated by a retired dentist who came to me for a consultation after having worked during the last years without sufficient eye protection.

3) In *yellow illumination* the perception of *blue pigment colors* is weakened, making all blue-painted objects disappear. Because of high luminosity, low pressure Sodium-lamps with the yellow illumination are widely used in road illumination, but these can distort color vision.

Besides their efficiency as light sources, low-pressure Sodium-light lamps produce a strict monochromatic yellow light—that is, containing only one single wavelength (589 nm). There is no reflection of blue pigment colors, which all appear as invisible dark surfaces[6]. In the large railway station for freights wagons at Alnabru, Oslo, the entire area was illuminated by monochromatic yellow light. This created the striking situation of engines and employees in their blue uniforms being invisible while their faces appeared as ghostly visages. When it comes to reflecting surfaces, we are all blue blind, while on the contrary our sensitivity to blue *light* is good (making it a good choice for emergency vehicles).

4) A special form of *blue blindness* exists as a *normal phenomenon.* In a restricted, minimal point in the central retina, the human eye is totally blue-blind. This can be demonstrated when looking at a distant object. Here a small, blue object cannot be seen when looking straight at it, but can be seen when looking at it from a little to the side. On the contrary, a red object is seen clearest by direct focusing.

An example from the First World War illustrates how dramatic this can be. French soldiers were wearing red caps (figure 20), and a high number of soldiers were shot through the head as soon as they looked out above the trench. They were ordered to use blue hats, and the incidence of being shot was markedly reduced. As the best perception of blue is a little outside the focus point (about two degrees from the center), the shooter's sight will be imprecise, and the shot will miss. In addition, the blue impulses are mediated slower than the green and red impulses in the visual system; also, their localization in the retina is less precise.

5) Unnatural colors, *chromatopsias,* are experienced by some people under special conditions. Chromatopsia is an abnormal state where the surroundings are seen in a certain color tint. It can occur when there is a distortion of the retina's equilibrium, as is seen occasionally after an

6 In order to avoid the unnatural and half magic feeling in the urban landscape, the City of Oslo decided to change the yellow lights to white lights in the town center.

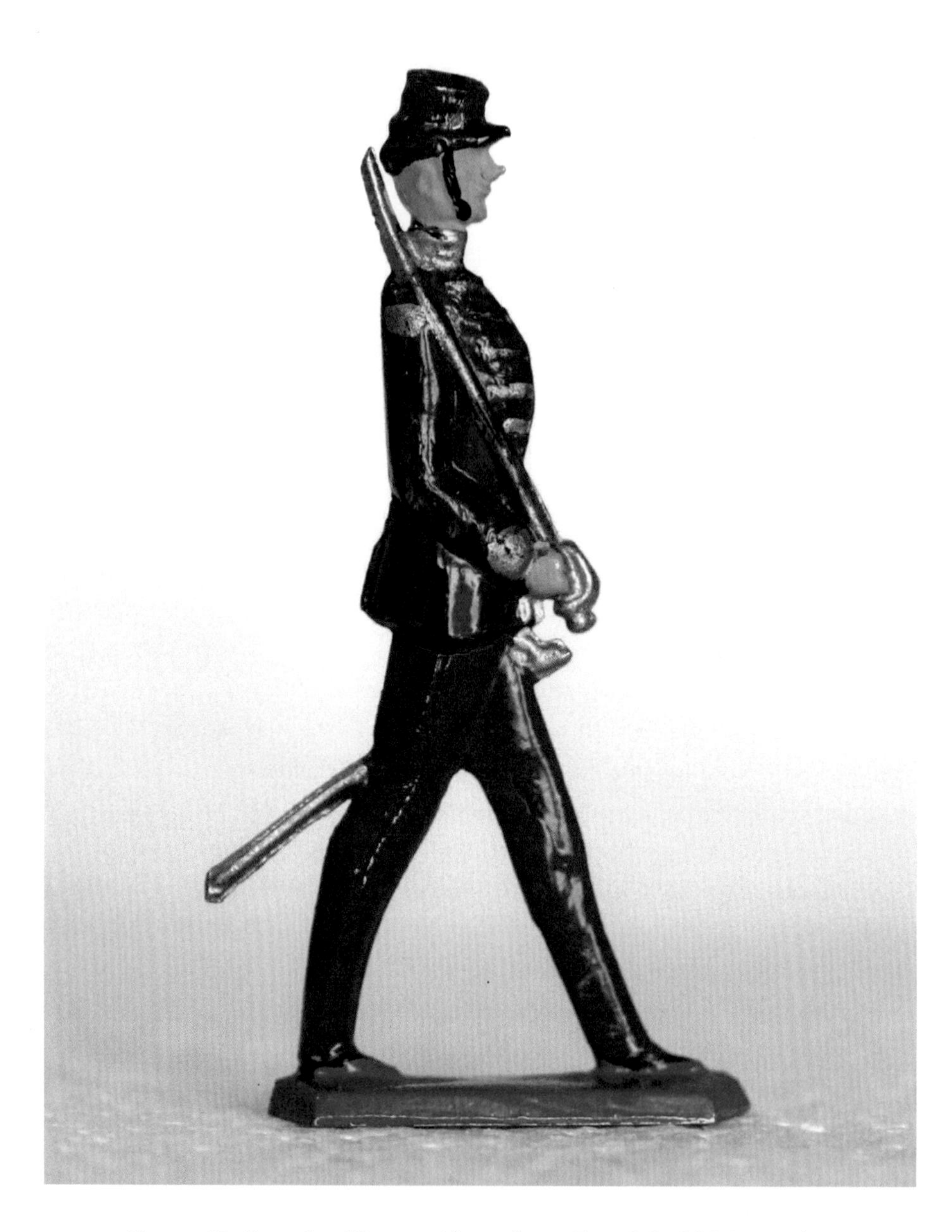

Figure 20. French officer uniform from First World War with a "kepi" in bright red. Pewter soldier in true copy (Knutsen 2000).

eye operation or in connection with the use of medicine. Most usual is "red-vision" (erythropsia). Chromatopsia can make its appearance after exposure to very strong light and especially where the pupil is dilated. Several medications can provoke chromatopsia. Digitalis can cause "green-vision"(chloropsia) and "yellow vision" (xanthopsia). As a rule, chromatopsia is temporary. Even though it causes anxiety, it does not result in visual loss or reduced color vision. "Yellow-vision" (xanthopsia) has been suspected in the great painter Vincent van Gogh (Marmor 2009) who in a period had used digitalis as well as absinthe. Absinthe was a common part of social, bohemian and artistic life in Pàris in the late nineteenth and early twentieth century, and used by several artists.

6) Hallucinations with colors.

One 85-year-old lady came to see me with macular degeneration and impaired vision. She sometimes noticed that she could see flowers of vivid colors on her walls, although there were no such motifs in color on her wallpaper. In earlier year, she had been much occupied with flowers. A color vision examination revealed that she had a blue-yellow color defect. However, this could not explain her thrilling experience with colored flowers. Another lady told that she could clearly see a group of children sitting on the floor in her home, although she knew no children were present.

The phenomena is an example of a peculiar neurological condition known as *Charles Bonnet's syndrome.* The patients with this disturbance have a disorder somewhere in the visual apparatus, the eye or in the brain, causing blindness or partial blindness.

V.S. Ramachandran described this condition in *Phantoms in the Brain* (Ramachandran 2005). He thinks the condition is rather common and can appear in patients having severe vision damage (for instance from glaucoma or retinal degeneration). There can be disturbance on the same level as other "phantom-phenomena," such what can be experienced when somebody is feeling pain in body parts that are amputated. Oddly enough, the disorder is not much known among doctors, probably because the patients are reserved in telling about their experience in order not to be considered "crazy."

7) Other false experiences of colors are described as *"synaestesia,"* when one type of perception releases sensations in other sensing systems. They are reported by some individuals provoked by certain stimuli such as written or spoken numbers, smells, scraping noise or melodies. They are quite seldom, but still a real phenomenon that is difficult to explain (Ramachandran 2011). Oliver Sacks tells about a girl with impaired vision from childhood whose intense synaestesia instantly triggered colors; for example, number 4 was gold and 5 light green. Days of the week, as well as months of the year, had their colors, too (Sacks 2010).

Such sensation of vivid colors released by listening to music is reported by some musicians (as will be referred to later on).

# CHAPTER 8: SOME ADVANTAGES OF COLOR BLINDNESS

Color blindness under primitive conditions would seem to be a disadvantage in the struggle for life. Many have speculated whether color blindness has influenced human development or whether the frequency of color blindness disadvantages in certain populations (Pickford 1965).

Observations in animal life have complicated the picture. In a study by A.D. Melin and colleagues, monkeys with severe red-green color deficiency were shown to be more effective in discovering and catching camouflaged insects than monkeys with normal color vision (Melin 2007).

*Can good color vision give a disadvantage?*

Sometimes normally sighted people fall short in endeavors to find hidden things in environments with an abundance of colors, where color blind people can easily see the hidden things. This fact is being used by the military, among other organizations. The contours of cannons, tanks, and other materiel are hidden under camouflage nets with strong colors in crisscross, irregular patterns. The hidden objects, however, are seen much easier by color blind persons who are not confused by the colors. During the Second World War, the British Royal Air Force picked out color blind persons to be sent in airplanes to identify camouflaged positions behind enemy lines.

*Can color blind people see black-white contrasts better than the normally sighted?*

There is no documentation that contrasts are better seen by the color blind than by other people, even though, theoretically, the more homogeneous cone mosaic in the retina of the color blind might facilitate contrast-perception. Yet sharpshooters are not infrequently color blind. In an exceptional case of acquired total color blindness, described by Oliver Sacks, the extraordinary loss of color vision brought about a marked sharpening of visual acuity (Sacks 1995).

*Does color blindness influence night vision?*

A study of S. Verhulst and F.W.Maes in the University of Groningen, the Netherlands reported that color blind men have a better visual ability than the color normal during scotopic conditions— i.e., during weak lighting at night. In this connection, color blindness is not necessarily a defect, but a benefit (Verhulst 1998).

*Can the color blind distinguish color nuances?*

Lack of ability to differentiate between nuances of color shades, is often associated with color blindness, but this is not always the case. Actually, some color blind people have a greater ability to discriminate color tints in parts of the color circle than people with normal sight. Paradoxically, this happens in just the parts of the color circle where the color blind's perception of color hues is especially weak (the green and red areas). Pitt's law expresses this (in people with color vision deficiency the ability to discriminate wavelength differences is best where the color saturation is poorest). The almost scary sensitivity to wavelength differences demonstrated by some color-defectives people is well known. Arthur Linksz, in *An Essay on Color Vision*, writes about textile dealers who can be a "terror" for salesmen, because they see better than the salesmen the finer hue differences in the consignments (Linksz 1964).

# CHAPTER 9: COMMUNICATION WITH COLORS

More thoughtful use of color messages can help to transmit information to persons with divergent color vision.

Colors are widely used in all sorts of circumstance—and often without thought or consideration. In a school, when young students are taught, for example, the difference between vowels and consonants, a teacher might have the idea to write the vowels with red chalk and the consonants with green chalk. Some pupils, not able to differentiate between vowels and consonants, might have the feeling of being stupid. In geography, mountains might be illustrated with brown colors and lowlands with green. But, again, there are those who are made to feel stupid by missing the clues. Using colors to clarify and explain things outside the classroom is equally unsuccessful. In a skiing competition where colored ribbons were used to show the direction of the ski track (mostly ribbons in red and pink attached to the green spruce trees), red-green defective competitors became confused. These are unfortunate colors to use when fairness is important to maintain.

## MISUSE OF COLORS

In daily life, good color vision is often taken for granted. Color is misused when the differences among people are not taken into consideration. For example, black printing of letters and numbers on red paper is commonly used for messages and warnings. This is particularly unfortunate for red-blind and red-weak people (the protanes), who see red surfaces as more or less grey and as very dark. Imagine reading black letters on a red background (figure 21).

Among other unfortunate combinations are traffic signs warning "No Parking" and "No Stopping" where the colors used are dull blue and red. As we have seen, red is usually a desaturated color for many color blind, it is perceived as nearly gray. Dull blue may be difficult to determine in bad lighting. So, for some individuals, differentiation between the two traffic signs can be very difficult or impossible, as was pointed out by a color blind man who complained of his trouble in a letter to the editor in a weekly journal in Oslo. (He was asked to come to our clinic and proved to be a protanope):

"Concerning writing on colored background - have a look on the bank giro transfer forms - the text is nearly unreadable for a color weak person. Extra lighting and a magnifying glass are required. Journals, magazines, periodicals, travel catalogs – all continue to use more colors on pages with letters in special colors, making it difficult to understand. And I should include the traffic sign "No Stopping Any Time." Red cross on dark blue background. Impossible to see! I have to climb onto the mast or ask a pedestrian whether there is a cross or a line".

Another unfortunate example is a stamp from the Norwegian Post Office in 1989 showing the value in red on a green background. A color blind person would not be able to see the value of the stamp, as pointed out in another letter to the editor:

"It is an unreasonable discrimination of this considerable minority when the post office distributes a 5-kroner stamp - the world championship 89 - showing the mark printed in red on a green background, making it impossible for the color blind to see the value of the stamp."

a)
In children with squinting eye the binocular vision is disturbed. The eye in
the deviating position is not in proper use, and a reduction of the visual
ability may be the result. Usually the parents are not aware of the visual
weakening of the child's eye as the other eye is still good.
In order to cure or prevent visual weakening, the best eye is occluded
and the child is forced to use her weakened and squinting eye.
It is usually practiced to change the covering between the two eyes.
The child should always have one eye covered, if nothing else has been
agreed.
b)
c)
Verdensmesterskapet '89
7
Norge
5.00
1989
Anisdahl

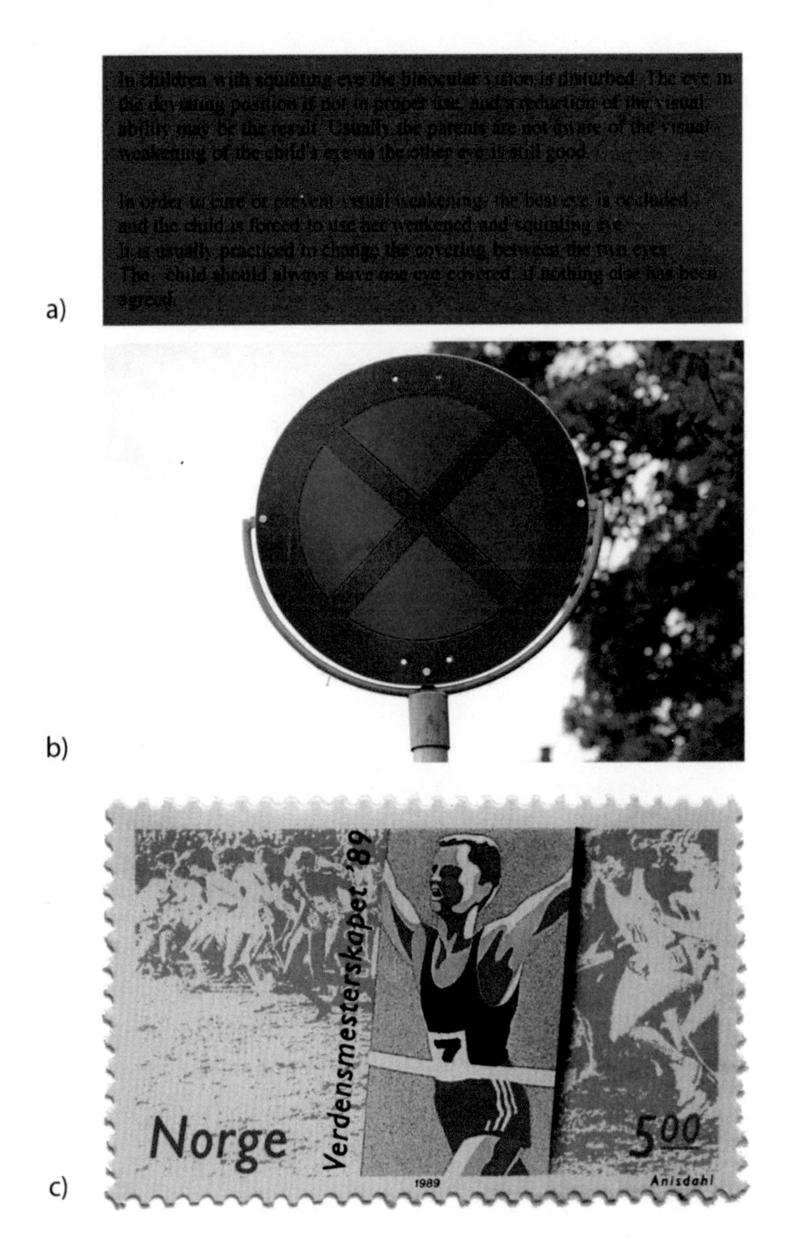

Figure 21. Examples of unfortunate color combinations for color blind persons: a) black writing on a red background, b) "No Parking Anytime" traffic sign, c) Old stamp with red value printed on a green area.

A journalist whom I diagnosed as a "red blind" (protanope) told a funny story about a soccer game. His favorite team was playing in green costumes, the other team in orange. "It was highly confusing," he began. "Twenty men in the same costumes were running aimlessly between two goalkeepers. Some defense players hurled the ball toward their own goal. The team members tackled each other violently and hard. The referee blew randomly for offside, free kicks, corners, and goals." (Henmo 2010).

Among other awkward situations are mistakes about toilets being occupied or not—on trains or airplanes, since red and green are commonly used to indicate whether the stalls are occupied or vacant.

The protanope reader who wrote a letter to the editor wondered at the attitude of the designers. "Isn't the purpose of colors on printed matters to make the message clearer? Journals and brochures of all kinds continuously increase their use of colors on the pages and letters, of which many are incomprehensible.." He added a rhetorical deep sigh: "In those cases it must really be possible for designers and color advisers to consult any color blind person, who will be able to say whether the printing matter is legible or not.."

## APPROPRIATE USE OF COLORS

By choosing colors for presentations in order to making things clearer, due consideration should be paid to the differences among us. Impairment of the red-green color sense, as is shown in the Farnsworth iso-color diagram (figure 12), implies certain confusing mistakes. The protane defectives confuse colors along the axis red - gray - blue-green and the deutanes along the axis red-purple - gray - green, but never across the confusion axes. Choosing colors across the main confusion axes can prevent problems for many color defective people. Such pairs of colors can be purple and purple-blue versus yellow and yellow-green or blue and blue-purple versus yellow and yellow-red.

For many partially sighted people good contrasts are important. Use of appropriate colors will increase contrast perception. When the authorities decided to change the color of the traffic poles in the city of Stockholm to a soft, mossy color instead of yellow, a wave of protests came from the union of the visually impaired. (Melander 1997). Yellow is a good and clear color and can also be easily seen by red-green defective people. A red-green blind colleague (and friend of mine) expressed his enthusiasm when he came to Sweden and found the post boxes painted in yellow, in contrast to the red post boxes in Norway!

For contrast perception in general, black writing on yellow surface has proved to deliver maximum clarity. In the same way, yellow middle part lines on roads are more easily seen than white lines. Therefore many road signs have been changed to black against yellow.

The physicists Thorstein Seim and Arne Valberg have studied how partially sighted persons perceive contrasts. They found that the use of one color together with a grey or white surface boosted the contrast perception, compared with black-white contrast. Their study also showed that the same good contrast perception was not achieved when two colors were used (Seim 1993).

A more conscious use of colors against neutral surfaces will enable more visually handicapped people to orient themselves in surroundings. In rehabilitation, medical professionals should know about the color vision of their clients to learn how to compensate for visual loss.

# CHAPTER 10: KEEPING PEOPLE SAFE

After it became clear that deficient color vision was a vocational risk on railways and at sea, the Great North Railway Company in Britain in about 1853 decided on a color vision standard. France followed in about 1858. The Swedish professor Alaric Frithiof Holmgren pleaded most eagerly for a standard after a great railway accident at Lagerlunda, Sweden, in 1875. He was convinced that the accident arose from an engineer with deficient color vision, and he persuaded the Swedish Railways and the Swedish Royal Navy to demand that officers and employees have normal color vision. Franz Cornelis Donders, the well known professor of physiology in Utrecht Netherlands, introduced his lantern test in 1877 for this purpose. (Ironically, Holmgren's assumption that defective color vision caused the Lagerlunda train collision was wrong. A.J. Vingrys and B.L. Cole, in their study in 1988 postulated that no train accidents in history can be attributed to deficient color vision (Vingrys 1988). But the Lagerlunda accident succeeded in establishing color-vision screening for railway employees, and the lantern test was adopted by railway systems in many countries.

## IN ROAD TRAFFIC

The approach taken for railways has not been mirrored for roadways. Red and green signal lights have a long legacy, with the position of the signal lights standardized—red on top and green below. One can ask why the traffic lights should absolutely depend on the use of red and green colors since red-green color vision defects are so commonly found. For instance, why not use blue and yellow or orange? The answer is that blue is not very suitable because the color penetrates poorly in haze and mist and has limited carrying capacity at a distance. Yellow and orange lights can seem rather colorless (desaturated). The luminous intensity in old lanterns used at sea was rather low, so filters transmitting more yellow green were used to increase their efficiency. (Modern signal lights are more powerful, with the green nearer to blue-green.)

So red and green remain the standard, despite that traffic lights can be misinterpreted by drivers with color-vision deficiency and despite that normal color vision is not required for driving cars, trucks, buses, and taxis. Nevertheless, one cannot ignore the possibility that traffic lights can be misinterpreted by color defective persons. Therefore, defective color vision is still a risk factor in driving (Cole 1997). However, this seems to be a risk most communities are willing to take.

This risk increases when traffic lights are seen separately, as when a single red or green light is positioned above a lane. A color blind man once told me that he preferred to bring his wife with him when driving with such signals.

It would benefit all communities if color vision were routinely tested as part of medical examinations. Drivers should learn about type and degree of a possible color vision defect. For example, a "red blind" person cannot be expected to see red traffic lights at a distance, and information written in black on red surface would be impossible to read.

## SAFETY PRECAUTION

Fast and precise recognition of warning colors (red, green and yellow) is particularly important in ensuring safety at sea, on the rails, and in the air. Seeing colors in a test situation, of course, is different from seeing the in emergency situations, such as in rough weather and bad visibility, especially since a failure of vision might be accompanied by things like skidding brakes, falling objects, onrushing vehicles, or information signs that may or may not be working. Fatal decisions can be taken when there is doubt about colors seen. Therefore, hesitations and uncertain answers during a color-vision test must be noted. White and yellow must also be understood immediately and correctly and should not be confused with green, red, or blue for instance. A quite common deficiency among partly color blind persons is the *falsely increased color contrast sensitivity* mentioned earlier. This can be important in situations with rapidly changing signal lights, which is often the case for engine drivers or speedboat sailors.

## PROFESSIONAL SECURITY REQUIREMENTS

In every country, standards have been established for checking the vision of employees who must be able to assess colored signs. In railways, normal color vision is generally required for all personnel operating trains (engine drivers and conductors) and personnel employed on the line. Tram drivers must also produce evidence of normal color vision. Bus drivers often don't need documentation of color vision as distinct from train personnel.

Normal color vision is demanded for sailors working at "the helm and the look- out." This includes navigators of ferry boats. But color vision is not required for those working in the engine room or in the galley. Since on modern ships a rotation principle holds that every sailor must be able to perform different kinds of work, it is now common to require documentation of normal color vision even for the engineers. Amateurs sailing big boats and yachts are also required to have normal color vision.

On the whole, navy rules mirror those of the merchant navy. In general, all the applicants to the naval academy and the naval training corps are required to document normal color vision. The applicants must be able to distinguish between red and green signal lights under ordinary conditions.

In the coastal artillery, red and green colored lights are important markers when firing and as signals during hand-to-hand combat. Here officers must also be able to identify yellow signal lights, which are used in modern mountain forts connected with protection against gas and radiation.

In aviation pilots and navigators must have normal color vision. Testing and acceptance of pilots in several countries is entrusted to special medical committees. In Norway, the Civil Aviation Authority uses the Holmes-Wright's color lantern and requires perfect performance. Normal color vision is demanded for hobby pilots. Amateurs who do not pass the lantern test are granted limited licenses for flying only in daylight.

## THE PAPI SYSTEM

People with the mildest degree of color-vision deficiency are usually able to interpret color signals satisfactorily. However, is it safe to also include them as aviation personnel?

This question was posed in 2009 by the English and American authors John Barbur, Sally Evans, and Nelda Milbum, in their study "Minimum Color Vision Requirements for Professional Flight Crew. Recommendations for New Color Vision Standards." (J. E. Barbur 2009).

The study reported that people with minimal color deficiencies often fail the most sensitive color-vision tests. The great majority of them are therefore prevented from becoming pilots, although many may well be able to perform critical safety tasks.

Which are the most important safety-critical, color-related tasks for pilots? The visual task analysis identified landing procedures as the most important part of a flight. And colors are the only clue used in he standard system for landing, the "Precision Approach Path Indicator" (PAPI). To ensure that an approaching airplane is at the correct level of altitude, the PAPI landing system uses a signaling system of four lights, two of which are white and two of which are red, when the airplane is at correct level. Any pilot seeing more than two white lights would assume a plane to be "too high"; and a pilot seeing more than two red lights would assume a plane to be "too low." Obviously, the ability to distinguish between red and white lights is critical.

For testing applicants, a true copy of an airport's installation and a PAPI simulator are used. Candidates are accepted for service when they correctly identify a series of lights of a great variety of red and white lights.

## THE CAD TEST

A new developed color vision test, the color assessment & diagnosis test (CAD test), which was developed by a team working with John Barbur from the Applied Vision Research Center in London, has shown to be very accurate in identifying the type and severity of one's color blindness. In the test the subject's task is to report the direction of motion of a colored square on a gray square background with dynamic changing luminance. The test is especially important in aviation medicine in order to identify limits for acceptance of colorblind pilot applicants, but it's also a valuable test for identifying diagnosis and degree of color defect in other connections, especially for following the development of acquired color vision defects (Barbur 2012).

## JUDGING SIGNAL LIGHTS AT SEA

Among anomalous trichromats, who cositute 70 percent of the color blind population, individuals vary from those with nearly normal color vision to those whose deficiencies compare to dichromats. Jo Ann Kinney and colleagues at the Naval Submarine Medical Research Laboratory in Connecticut carried out realistic tests on a dark beach where different types of light could be seen from ships that were located at different distances from the beach. The experiment was carried out in order to learn how well people with different types of color deficiency and those with normal vision were able to identify colored signals in their natural surroundings. The normally sighted people carried out the job satisfactorily, while the people with color-vision deficiency performed relatively poorly. As would be expected, men with minor defects did better than those with greater defects. However, in each category, from mild to severe defects, and for protane as well as deutane, some had a perfect score on the practical tests (Kinney 1979). This shows that it is difficult to predict the performance of color defectives in practical situations.

Recognition of red, green, and white colored lights in the night was tested with distances of one, two, and three miles from the beach (10, 5, and 3 arc seconds). With red light, the results were relatively good. More errors came when the light changed to white or green. There was a marked worsening with increasing distance. For the protanes (red defectives), identification of green and white was poor, even at a short distance. Most commonly, green signals were mistaken for white and vice versa. For people with color-vision deficiency there were great individual differences within each category of defect. The greatest surprise was noticed for the deutanes (green defectives). An important result from the study was the realization that one could not predict with certainty which men would do well in real-life situations and who would not. Protanes (red defectives) had poorer scores than the deutanes. A great deal of the errors was due to their inability to see the lights at a long distance. Decreased brightness perception of the red signals (the luminosity loss) for protanomalous and protanopes is well known. However, confusing green and white was a common error.

For all types of color-deficiencies, the variations in the error scores were not correlated with intelligence, motivation or experience.

## SEEING FIRE

Active firemen constitute an especially vulnerable group for whom identification of fresh flames as well as fire within heavy smoke is vital. This was dramatically demonstrated during the 2010 conflagrations in Australia (Dain 2003). Under the Australian National Commercial Drivers regulations, crewmen who extinguish fires are tested for or must report any possible color-vision defects. Protane defectives (the red deficient) are excluded.

Color is an important warning in helping to discover smoke and flames. Fire fighters must be able to locate and identify red fire trucks, and they must be able to make out their colleagues among green and brown vegetation. Among firemen who perished in the Australian wildfires of 2010, a common cause was the loss of visual contact with the fire trucks and the service cars (which had the standard colors of red and white).

# CHAPTER 11: MANAGING SCHOOL AND WORK

Early examination of color vision in children can prevent misunderstandings in elementary school as well as frustrations later in life.

## ELEMENTARY SCHOOL

When a child starts school, he or she should have a a color vision examination. Such routine screenings take little time and are extremely important to the child, but also to teachers. Ideally, adults should be aware of possible handicaps early on before a child starts school. The first days of school should be a happy occasion that fosters a  positive attitude to school. By contrast, undiscovered handicaps can bring about frustrations, errors, and sometimes reproach, resulting in confusion and unpleasant feelings.

Roswell Gallagher and Constance Gallagher point out that problem in an article in *Archives of Ophthalmology* (Gallagher 1964). Visual and hearing deviations, including color-vision deficiency, should be explained to the student  as well as to parents and the teacher. Maureen Neitz and Jay Neitz, based in Wisconsin, have designed a "mass screening test" that makes it possible to test school children quickly and reliably, using a previously calibrated paper-and-pencil test (Neitz 2001). Thousands of copies of the test were produced and distributed to schools in Wisconsin. Pupils aged four to twelve years used their pencils to trace figures they saw in illustration charts. Some charts were of the "vanishing type" (including symbols which would be invisible to the children with color-vision deficiency) and others of the "transformation type" (figures which would be identified differently by children with normal vision and those with color-vision deficiency).

## HIGH SCHOOL, UNIVERSITY, AND VOCATIONAL STUDIES

Generally, color vision does not affect admission to secondary schools and universities in Western Europe and the United States. Other countries can be more restrictive—among them Japan, which once required normal color vision for entrance into high school and university. With an iron hand, color blind students were excluded until the 1990s. Then Japanese doctors petitioned for a policy similar to that in Western countries. Today, except for some instances involving training for positions in national security, even totally color blind students can generally be accepted for admission for university study. (This does not mean, however, that everybody can ignore color vision. Academic studies often need to be adapted for persons with divergent color vision.)

For instance, training institutions for the fishing and shipping trades in Norway are obliged to inform applicants that they are subject to certain requirements vis-à-vis various maritime licenses and color vision ability.

Vocational schools vary when it comes to color-vision regulations. Good color vision is required for electricians, as well as for those performing low-current work in which numerous color-coded cords are used. In addition, good color vision is generally required for vocational training of textile workers and furniture upholsterers.

In some countries, standards have been requested for certain unusual occupations—such as diamond cutters and seed classifiers. Special tests have been designed for such kind of work by private enterprises (like the Munsell Color Company).

## OTHER PROFESSIONAL SPHERES

Many professions require that good color vision be documented even when it is not vitally important. The army in some countries demands color-vision tests for admission to officer candidate schools, army signal corps, and weapons-technology units, presumably to insure against misunderstandings. Entrance into police ranks usually requires normal color vision.

For physicians, no demands about color vision exist either for admission to medical school or for license to practice. However, color vision can still be important: surgeons must differentiate between bile ducts and blood vessels; physicians using endoscopy or pathologists using microscopic samples need uncompromised visual acuity and color vision. Screening for color vision as part of admission to medical studies could be advantageous to the profession, and has been asked for (Spalding 1997), (Hem 2004). Such screening is already in place for maritime medical practitioners who screen sailors for acceptance in the Norwegian merchant fleet; they must meet a requirement of normal color vision.

Dentists and dental technicians need good color vision for precise evaluation of the color of teeth and dental crowns as well as color abnormalities in the mouth. But there are no formal demands for normal color vision either.

One can find a wide range of requirements for documentation of normal color vision for a diversity of jobs. Richmond Products - dealers of ophthalmic instruments- has compiled a list of 100 jobs where normal color vision is needed. This, however, reflects exaggerated caution and is based on scanty knowledge of color-vision defects. In fairness, color-vision requirements should be proportionate to the tasks in any articular position.

# CHAPTER 12: COMPENSATION AND TREATMENT

The idea of being able to eliminate color blindness by using filters or special glasses is alluring, especially when it comes to seeing signal lights. Colored filters can indeed make certain colors appear clearer. They can appear with greater brightness while other colors can appear softened. Colored filters can change mutual brightness—in other words, some colors seem brighter and others softer. This indeed enhances the ability to identify colors[7].

> Color blindness cannot be eliminated, but the characteristics of some colors can be heightened, allowing for easier identification of colors.

Early experiments with colored filters met some success. A report by the physicist August Seebeck, in 1837, proposed using a red filter, then a

7 Colored filters are also used by people with normal color vision in order to increase color contrasts. For instance, ophthalmologists insert a green filter in their instruments to increase the contrasts and evaluate the fine vessels in the retina. By using so-called "red free" illumination, the vessels are made to appear as dark contours against a brighter background.

green filter, to evaluate colors when there was a change of brightness (Sharpe 2001). Likewise, the famous physicist James Clerk Maxwell in 1855 tried out filters for identifying traffic lights, recognizing anatomical dyes and color-coded cables.

The use of colored filters has been resumed in recent years, among others by Robert Fletcher in London City University (Fletcher 1982). Magenta, red, and green filters are all used by people with color-vision deficiencies. In some cases, filters have proved useful, especially for sorting colored things. Likewise, colored filters have helped color blind people distinguish between red and green colors that they can otherwise scarcely distinguish.

The most popular filters are red "high pass" filters, magenta filters, and green filters. Some of these can fit into contact lenses or, as colored glass, inserted into eyeglasses on one side or both. Such filters are intended for special tasks, but they may have certain unfavorable effects, such as reduced luminance and visual acuity, distortion of the visual picture, and change of stereoscopic and depth vision.

Unfortunately, even a moderately dense red filter can be hazardous for car driving and aviation, especially at night. It can cause difficulty in estimating speed and it can reduce depth vision.

Colored filters are not suitable at sea and should not be used when at "helm and outlook." Regulations still require good color vision for navigation at sea and do not accept color filters as a compensation.

In the end, colored filters can yield partial improvement in discriminating colors but they contribute little, if anything, in real, practical situations. Even so, it can be said that, for instance, a magenta contact lens on one eye can be a supplement; patients can use it if they feel it gives them an advantage without being inconvenient. But its effect is not enough for safety at work. A practical arrangement is to have filters handy, placing them in front of the eye when a color is in doubt. Some people have found it useful to attach red and green strips to the upper part of the lenses of their eyeglasses (Sharpe 2001).

Some people have eagerly sought other remedies, trying various medicines and high doses of vitamins to "cure" color blindness or avoid errors in color vision tests. Some have tried pure charlatan treatments, such as the injection of extracts from snakes, the overheating of the eyes, or electrical shocks. One nearly desperate aviation recruit asked about the possibility of having new eyes transplanted!

> *What seems absurd may not be entirely unthinkable. A sensational experiment recently carried out on monkeys by Mancuso and coworkers—and published in 2009 in Nature—demonstrates that it is possible to cure color blindness by gene therapy. Two adult monkeys, red-green blind from birth, obtained full color vision following the injection of gene material into their retina. Thus, a trichromatic color vision was established in place of their original dichromatic vision* (Mancuso 2009). *What is not possible today, may perhaps come into use for treating color blindness in the future.*

Colored filters do not change the fact that the color-vision defect is still present. They only change the condition under which the colors are seen. Some people go astray and believe that their color vision has been improved, since they become able to read the figures as in the Ishihara test. A magenta filter may allow an examinee to see many of the figures in the test. But the Ishihara test is designed for a certain type of illumination (daylight or lamps with daylight quality). If the illumination is wrong, the test is worthless. Using filters is tantamount to a drastic change of illumination, and so it makes the test useless. Likewise, the use of filters will change the settings in the anomaloscope where the proportion of red and green qualities (expressed by the green-red quotient) is changed. For instance, the green-red quotient can be falsely lowered by using green sunglasses. Nevertheless, colored filters *can* be useful in certain situations to distinguish between colors, since some colors will appear brighter while others will appear darker. But this is not valid for all situations.

One would expect a red filter would make a red surface shine through with an even more colorful tint. However, the result is the opposite. When seen through the red filter, the red surface will appear quite pale, even colorless, or white. The phenomenon has been named after the mathematical genius, Gaspard Monge, who presented it at a lecture in Paris in 1789 just before the revolution. In his 2005 survey, John Mollon called the phenomenon "the paradox of Monge." (Mollon 2006). Monge's explanation has stood as the first description of the phenomenon "colors' constancy." Colors are not only a result of the wavelengths of the light reaching the retina. The colors are processed by impulses in the brain which take into account the surroundings under which the colors are seen.

Using color filters is not suitable for seeing color *hue* better, but is suitable for seeing color *brightness* better.

Quite another principle in compensating for color blindness is now introduced with color scanners modified for use as a remedy for helping partially sighted and blind persons to identify colors. Such a scanner is available, among others, by the firm Adaptor as a portable instrument called the Colorino Color Indicator. With the instrument, one can read whether a signal from a surface is red or green. (For instance, in the newspaper company VG, color scanners have been introduced to make visually handicaped persons able to read the red and green codes used in the doors for access to the offices).

# V: COLOR BLINDNESS AND ART

# CHAPTER 13: DEVIANT COLOR VISION IN ART

Colors have a central position in the visual arts, enhancing creative expression. Artists want their messages to reach an audience, but if the perception of colors differs greatly from the artist to the receiver, the message will be lost. What the spectator takes as disturbing—or even deviant—might be an intentional effort by the artist to use color in a way that is out of the ordinary. It can be risky to draw conclusions about an artist's color vision from his paintings.

*When Edward Munch's paintings in the University assembly hall were presented in 1914, Hjalmar Schiøtz, the famous Norwegian ophthalmologist, doubted the color vision of the artist. During the discussions in the academic council about the decoration in the assembly hall, Schiøtz voted against Munch's paintings on the grounds that Munch probably was color blind. Schiøtz expressed his wish to examine Munch's color vision* (Johansen 1978). *As far as anyone knows, no one ever examined Munch's color vision. However, there is no reason to doubt that Munch's color vision was normal.*

Munch broke with the conventions of painting, so while some people reacted to his pictures with enthusiasm, others thought the pictures showed his flawed understanding and ability.The latter group pronounced the work hideous and deviant.[8]

---

8 An exception was Arnulf Øverland,, a young author who said that Munch's "laurel wreath cannot be talked away".

Munch is not the only ground-breaking painter who has been suspected of being color blind. Several authors have pointed out that certain painters "must" be color blind. However, in general, no examination of the artists' color vision has been carried out. Whether shrewd or unjustified, over the years conclusions have been drawn based on indications, not evidence.

That color vision is important for pictorial artists is, however, unquestionable. So for those wanting to make art their career, color-vision deficiencies can pose problems. One young man who came to my office wanting a color-vision examination told me that he had started his training for painting by correspondence. It appeared that he had a red-green color vision defect, for on one occasion he had painted the sky violet instead of blue. He came to realize that following his ambition as a painter might prove problematical and discontinued his training.

## HOW CAN THE INFLUENCE OF COLOR VISION AMONG ARTISTS BE ESTIMATED?

Certainly some great artists have persisted even though they did not have normal color vision. In certain cases an artist can, regardless of his color vision, evoke general admiration for his personal and characteristic style.

Charles Merion, a well known artist in the 19th century, was color blind, cofirmed by his doctor. Also Paul Henry, praised as the finest Irish painter in the last century, had a total red-green color blindness ascertained by his doctor, though it was a hidden secret during his lifetime (Marmor 2009).

And for some painters with known color-vision defects, of varied degrees, the deficiency did not necessarily show in their pictures. Sven Larsson, in his book "The Artist's Eye," tells about the Swedish painter Torsten Palm, who was praised as an exquisite landscape painter. Both he and his brother were known to be color blind. He was referred to as "the green-blind friend," though he called himself the "gray painter." He preferred neutral, gray nuances and his fine coloring was appreciated by many (Larsson 1965).

## WHICH ELEMENTS IN A PAINTER'S PRODUCTION CAN REVEAL A COLOR-VISION DEFECT?

The selection of colors used in paintings does not automatically lead to a diagnosis of a painter's color vision. Some criteria have, however, been ascribed as more significant than others:

1 Preference for gray tints in the painting;
2 Choosing dominating contrasts in yellow and blue colors;
3 Use of "wrong" colors;
4 Prevalence of heavily colored shadows;
5 Infrequency of color nuances.

**Criterion** 1. The fact that some artists have renounced using high color content in their paintings, preferring to paint in shades of gray and black, is said to indicate color deficiency. The paintings are said to have a striking poverty of clear colors but are rich in nuances among the few colors used. For the known color blind painters (among them Meryon and Henry), there was an inclination to use black and white in their paintings. Charles Meryon was an important artist in the 19th century. Even though that he realized his color vision defect in his early years. he still continued his artistic career. However, he often preferred beautiful black prints, in which one can see the graduation of shading. He realized that his congenital defect in color vision made work in oil too difficult. Only one oil painting with colors and one colored pastel are known from his production. He turned to printmaking where he had great success, like his most famous series of etching, "Scenes of old Paris" (Marmor 2009).

Brownish nuances were used with preference by John Constable, leading to a suspicion of deviant color vision, (see Larsson.) However, this was not supported in a color-vision evaluation. The Danish artist Vilhelm Hammershøi was called "the gray painter," but no information is available about his color vision. He is characterized as having a striking color perception "in a world of color not at all common with that of other painters." Speculation about color blindness was especially provoked because of the artist's subdued shades in a dominant, clayish gray. Penetrating "analysis" is done on the basis of Hammershøi's paintings, but without any reference to the examination of color vision.

The tendency to paint with achromatic colors (black and white or gray-scale) occurs with many artists without suspecting of color vision dficiencies. Several artists in the minimalist tradition have clearly used monochromatic colors. The American painter Ad Reinhardt pared paintings to its bare essentials and was known for his "black paintings" that varied very little in tone. The Norwegian painter Kåre Tveter favored strong contrasting colors in his earlier years, but in his later years preferred very diffuse shades dominated by gray, yet also with images with sharp contrasts in black and white. The contemporary artist Jan Groth paints minimalistic lines in black and white.

**Criterion 2.** Another sign of color-vision defect is a preference for blue and yellow over green and red hues. Michael Marmor and James Ravin in their book "The Artist's Eyes" tell of a totally red-green blind painter, *Paul Henry*, whose portrayal of the blue mountains, white cottages and the silver-white clouds of the Irish landscape, showed a particular gift. In his first artistic years, he had a fondness for drawings, but later on for painting using blue and yellow as dominating colors. He preferred painting in early mornings when colors tended to be cool. Paul Henry was arguably the most important Irish painter of the twenties century, and his work was appreciated by many. He never mentioned his color deficiency in public, nor did he ever write about it. It was kept as a secret. Knowledge of his deficiency comes from his ophthalmologist, Dr. Beecher Sommervill-Large, who revealed the secret after Paul Henry's death.

R. W. Pickford examined several artists and noted that painters with severe color-vision defects avoid using red and green colors as contrast, preferring brightness contrasts and contrasts in yellow-blue. One color blind (protanope) artist stood out for his great skill in the use of color. He did not commit the expected blunders and was not willing to admit any defects in color vision (Pickford 1951).

Some famous painters are said to have been diagnosed with a color-vision defect. The Swedish ophthalmologist Gøsta Karpe, in an article in 1962, gave the French painter Fernand Léger as an example (Karpe 1962). The color composition and dominance of yellow and blue in Léger's paintings at an exhibition led the eye doctor J. Strebel to suspect that Léger had a color-vision defect. Strebel then had the opportunity to examine Léger and ascertained that the artist indeed had a red-green color defect. Sven Larsson, who attempted to verify the claim of color blindness in Léger, found no support for it in contemporary knowledge of the painter's use of color.[9] (Larsson 1965).

**Criterion 3.** Artists using unconventional colors (deemed "wrong") find that audiences may assume they have a color-vision defect. The bright, sparkling colors of Munch's painting of the sun—as well as other paintings in the University Assembly Hall in Oslo —led to a lot of criticism. But with the development of expressionism, such use of color became more common. Some artists deliberately began to use the "wrong" colors. The most extreme form arrived with the *fauvists*, a circle of painters at the beginning of 20th century who deliberately provoked by their use of wild colors and sharp contrasts. Critics labeled the painters "*fauve*" (French for wild or savage), but their use of color was entirely intentional and not an expression of defective color vision.

**Criterion 4.** The colored shadows used by some painters have been interpreted as signs of a color defect. When the German ophthalmologist Richard Liebreich, at an exhibition in London in 1872, noticed that some artists painted roofs and cows red on the well-lit side and green on the dark side, he drew the conclusion that the artists were red-green-blind. In Liebreich's schema, a naked child in the shadow would be painted green by the artist. In fact, any shadows painted in bright colors—in contrast to the illuminated sides of a subject—were thought to reveal color-vision defects (Larsson 1965).

As we have seen, bright colors can, in many color-defective people, evoke a contrast color that is complementary to the first color. This phenomenon is

9 Anomalous color vision, which can be diagnosed in the anomaloscope, may also include people with a mild degree of color defect. This, however, has little influence on their painting.

often particularly vivid in color weak people (anomalous trichromats) and is described as "falsely increased contrast sensitivity."

However, contrast sensitivity is a natural phenomenon that can also be expressed in the paintings of painters with normal color vision. The presentation of contrasting colored shadows does not, therefore, have to be a sign of defective color vision.

This phenomenon triggered a lively discussion in the Oslo Medical Society when *Munch* painted an old man with a green beard in his Aula picture *The History*. But one of the debaters said he had even seen a man in the students' park whose beard suddenly appeared green (Johansen 1978).

**Criterion** 5. The wealth of nuances in paintings, as well as the ability to produce the smallest change of hues, requires good color vision. The French ophthalmologist Philippe Lanthony in his book "The Painters' Eyes" writes: "There are things that the Daltonian (i.e. color blind person), even to a lesser degree, cannot do: the exact mix of colors, the subtle modulations of the tonalities. Their absence is in no way a sign of Daltonism, but rather their presence serves almost certainty to confirm that the color vision of the artist is normal."

This may be accurate for the greater part of the color-hue circle, but some individual red-green blind persons have a striking ability to evaluate green shades and to find matching colors in this part of the color circle. Despite their weak green perception, they may see a wide gamut of greens. (Remember Pitt's law, cited earlier: Color discrimination is at its best for people with color-vision deficiency where color perception is worst.) Likewise, the Swedish ophthalmologist Gøsta Karpe writes in an article that certain forms of so-called green blindness can be compatible with increased sensitivity to subtle nuances, which could conceivably be of value to painters (Karpe 1962).

As we have seen, the aforementioned "criteria" for color blindness in artists are without universal validity. Philippe Lanthony, who has carried out thorough art history studies, warns against drawing far-reaching conclusions about artists' color vision merely based on their production (Lanthony 1999).

## CATARACTS

Cataracts, the clouding of the lens that typically occurs in older years, leads to blurred and reduced vision. In addition, they can reduce color vision. This can have great consequences for painters.

The changes seen with cataracts are slow and gradual; likewise, changes to color vision because of cataracts does not show abrupt changes. The changes are often imperceptible. Cataract in a slight degree does not cause problems for color vision, but with increasing density and yellow coloring of the lens - yellowish or brownish coloring of the lens occurs not infrequently - blue and violet hues become less marked and more poorly distinguished.

In many patients developing cataracts, the blue-green, blue and violet hues appear weaker. But this transition is still imperceptible to most. Radiation in red, yellow and yellow-green light penetrates better than radiation in the blue end of the spectrum, and the world is gradually seen in a more yellowish hue. But still, the artist may recall colors and may be able to "look to his inner eye" when the tones of indigo-blue and blue have become weakened or absent. The artist often compensates by making the blue and violet colors too powerful. We see this especially in previous centuries, when it was usual to wait for the cataract to be "mature" before operating. Artists today experience less change in color perception, because cataracts are now operated on at a much earlier stage.

Another thing that contributes to the yellowing of vision with age is the macular pigment (the "yellow spot") in the center of the retina, which filters and gradually absorbs short-wave-length light. In this way, a more or less weakening of vision can occur in elderly artists.

Deterioration of color perception in pictorial artists can be noticed by a gradual change of coloring. In milder cataracts, no change in color processing takes place. When the deterioration of color perception happens little by little, the use of color, though unconsciously, changes over time. It results in an exaggeration of blue and purple in the pictures or, conversely, changing over to a weaker blue, or a warmer palette.

Many artists in old age like to paint in blue shades. Among the Swedish painters who painted in blue-violet shades in advanced age, Sven Larsson, in his book The Artist's Eye, mentions Prince Eugen, who had asked his friends to warn him when he started using stronger blue paint (Larsson 1965).

The English painter Mulready used more blue and purple in his later works (Charman 1976). It is likely that as blue became more muted, he compensated by using copious amounts of blue or, as another alternative, tended to use more exclusively red pigment that still had brilliance for him. A clearer change to red, orange, and yellow-green is demonstrated in Joseph Turner's work. An example of exaggeration of red is also seen with Auguste Renoir, whose palette reddened as he aged.

W.N. Charman and N.C. Evans made objective measurements of the pictures of the painter Georges Rouault over many years. They compared coloring from the early years with the paintings he produced after 70 years (Rouault painted until his death at 87 in 1958). His last works show a shift in colors suggestive of cataract. He painted with an overall reddish-yellow tone with rough strokes of paint. It has been recently demonstrated that little color was used from the short wavelength or blue end of the spectrum in contrast to that used in the pictures from the early years. However, the artist's eyes were not examined, so the conclusion that his lens became more yellow with age is just based on general knowledge.

In the case of Claude Monet, we have reliable information on the development of his cataract, because Philippe Lanthony made representative measurements of the artist's color palette from different periods in Monet's life (Lanthony 1999).

Monet was diagnosed with cataracts at the age of 71. He saw almost nothing with the right eye for several years, but he saw with his left eye and continued to paint until the cataract had progressed so far in the left eye that he could see no more than the largest letters on the vision board (visual acuity: 0.1). In an article in 1908, he described his struggle with colors in sad terms and he cut some of his canvases to shreds (Dietrichs 2008). Lanthony quotes Monet saying that he did not see the colors with the same intensity as before: "The red looks muddy to me, and the rose-colored is pale pink and colorless, and with the shades in between the weaker tones escape me. The delicate colored passages were no longer my affair."

Lanthony reviewed Monet's pictures, measuring individual colors in the pictures with reference to Munsell's atlas. He found that the cold colors dominate while the cataract was in the developing stage, while the warmer colors dominate in the later paintings. From one period to the other, a remarkable preponderance of the color line towards the yellow-green exists because of the cataract. He continued to have difficulties with subtle, delicate colors viewed up close. In 1922, he declared that he was no longer capable of making something of beauty. He destroyed several of his panels. With his best eye (the left - the right had been useless for many years) he could read only 20/200. In 1923, Monet underwent a two-stage cataract operation to his right eye. He was very disappointed by the operation, and he blamed the doctor. His left eye still contained a dense yellow-brown nuclear cataract. His color perception with the two eyes differed markedly. Violets and blues could stimulate the retina of his postoperative right eye, while these colors could not penetrate the cataract of his left eye. His world changed alternatively between too yellow and too blue. He began to destroy canvases from his preoperative period, and friends and family had to intervene to save many of the works. After the cataract surgery, he could not get accustomed to his new glasses with one thick lens which was necessary for his aphakic eye. Objects curved abnormally, and the colors were strange. However, the surgeon was satisfied and said that his vision at near might be considered nearly perfect. Still the artist remained discouraged and depressed, saying that painting is so difficult and a torture. His depressive mood improved by July 1925 when he stated that he had recovered his true vision nearly at a single stroke. The paintings from after the cataract surgery resemble his style of painting from 1917 or before (Marmor 2009).

After the cataract surgery in 1923, Monet's canvases suddenly returned to a preponderance of colder colors until his death in 1926.

We have thus seen that some painters use more purple and blue with age, perhaps to portray what they know and remember. The pictures will be more blue and violet than earlier, and may also reflect a more expressive form of painting. On the other hand, others such as Rouault and Monet use more warm shades.

Conversely, painters with an impressionistic way of painting, who strive for pure sense perception, will paint it more as it really looks to them. Because the perception of bluish hues in the scene diminishes with age, canvases show fewer blue tones and a warmer palette.

## THE EFFECT OF SURGERY

In earlier time, cataract surgery involved the removal of the lens without a new lens being inserted in the eye. This lens-less condition (aphakia) involved a more drastic effect on color vision than when either an artificial or a natural lens is present.

The effect of aphakia on color vision is diametrically opposed to that of cataract. There is first a sudden transition, and the patients are aware of this important abrupt change which they then has to adapt to. The operation also takes away the normal filter effect that results in short wavelength rays reaching the retina. The patient sees the color line completely modified and dominated by cool colors.

Lanthony found that shortly after surgery, Monet temporarily painted with a strong dominance of blue and violet shades. When Monet suddenly had his cataract removed, the eye that had been operated on, without a lens, perceived the colors as more towards the "colder" end. He regained a color perception that was more balanced and equal to his old feeling of colors.

It is interesting to go back and look at Monet's penchant for using warm tones during the development of his cataracts. Maybe he chose a palette of warm tones just because he was an impressionist, because what he saw were objects poor in blue and purple. He was more conscious of the real sensory impact and painted accordingly, while other artists who express their painting in the colors they remember, have a tendency to use the more powerful blues on the canvas. They lay the color on thick to get the tones in blue and purple. It's a big difference between what one really sees and what one reproduces in a painting from what it is more or less remembered.

## HOW DOES COLOR BLINDNESS INFLUENCE CHOICE OF ART FORM?

The number of color blind artists in the history of art is probably greater than we usually assume. If the color deficiency occurs in an extra mild degree, the artist would have no hindrance at all. Some may have mild color-deficiencies (mostly anomalous trichromats), which may or may not have been diagnosed and may or may not be known by the artist. The deficiency may have minimal consequences in the use of color. When color blindness is more pronounced, though, the art might have suffered.

Sven Larsson found the same frequency of color blindness in art schools, handicraft schools, and the community in general. Of 26 male students at an academy of fine arts, two were affected with color-perception defects (which matches the frequency in the population). The degree and type of color-vision defects were not stated, though. These students had not noticed any difficulty in their painting, reinforcing the idea that normal color vision is not an absolute requirement for painters.

Wolfgang Jaeger relates how Goethe had studied a color blind person's use of color by making a double set of a painting after directions from the person, a painter who was probably a protanope. Goethe designed a circular palette and then painted a landscape following the instructions of the color blind painter. Goethe used two methods, first duplicating the canvases of the painter and then painting spontaneously. In the resulting paintings, the sky was pink and the leaves yellow (Jaeger 1994).

Charles Meryon was a well-known 19th century artist in Paris who was clearly color blind according to indications and his own statement. He told: "Certain colors that are very different for everyone else, are all the same for me," He confused some colors, especially yellow and red paint when the paint was diluted with water. He could not distinguish between ripe strawberries and their leaves. On the palette he used red for yellow and pink for green; but he could distinguish carmine, gold, cobalt, and lapis lazuli, among other colors. Unfortunately for medical scholars, Meryon left few paintings behind. What survive of his work are mostly drawings in black chalk (Marmor 2009).

Psycho-physiologically, Daltonians have been shown to have no better contrast perception for achromatic shades than the normal person, but the great artists among them, undistracted by the play of colors in their world, learn to make full use of the contrasts.

Studying the choice of expression of color blind painters and their artistic development yields interesting information on the attitudes of color blind artists. Weak color vision can result in a greater interest in drawing than in painting.

Some color blind artists have switched from painting to other art forms like sculpture. Others often have a preference for sketching but less for colors. Phillipe Lanthony found that 17 out of 31 diagnosed Daltonians who were artists had chosen graphics (Lanthony 2001). Color blind painters who continue painting can avoid mistakes by arranging colors in unchanging order, naming the tubes, or using a reduced palette, among other strategies.

## ALIEN COLORS IN ART

A kind of alien colors are the chromatopsies which have been described earlier and arise from different causes, often intoxications. Vincent van Gogh had a striking use of yellow in his paintings. Marmor and Ravin referred to a long list of possible causes (Marmor 2009). One possible cause was kinin which had been used by van Gogh and is known to cause xanthopsia (yellow vision). Another explanation is that van Gogh's yellowish paintings may be caused by absinthe-induced xanthopsia. Absinthe was a drink that had been commonly used by van Gogh as well as by many artists at that time (Dietrichs 2008). It is therefore possible that van Gogh had experienced xanthopsia, but probably not as a continued phenomenon (sensations could be used by artists even if they had experienced strange sensations only for a short time).

Charles Bonnets syndrome may give rise to hallucinations with color (as referred to earlier). Strange sensation of colors may be connected with the phenomenon synaestesia where particular smells, names or numbers may elicit colors; so also with music.

## RELATION TO MUSIC

Colors have symbolic significance in other disciplines besides art—and the significance is often mysterious or speculative. However, some artists feel a special and strong connection between music and colors. The Russian painter Alexel von Jawlensky considered painting "visual music," where each color corresponded to an equivalent sound. He developed this idea into a series of abstract paintings that he called "Songs without Words." (The 20th-Century Art Book 1999).

An even closer link between music and colors existed for the French composer Olivier Messiaen. He had a remarkable ability to experience color and music simultaneously. He declared that certain timbral and rhythmic sequences promoted specific color perceptions. The critics even called him "*le fauviste en musique*" (a fauvist musician). Also the Russian composer Alexander Shrjabin vividly perceived color in conjunction with certain musical keys.

This additional or extra sense perception, termed *synesthesia*, is often related to music. Oliver Sacks gives a broad description of the phenomenon in his book *Musicophilia* (Sacks 2007). Synesthesia may also apply to taste, smell or numbers. Musicians who see colors together with music find it incomprehensible that others don't. So incomprehensible that they believe others must have some form of "color blindness." Color-music synesthesia is more common than we know about, probably because people do not spontaneously talk about it and doctors do not ask about it. Sacks counts it as a physiological phenomenon that can be based on an excess of neurological connections between the areas of the brain. V. S. Ramachandran asserts that synestesia is favoured by localization to nearby areas in the brain (Ramachandran 2011).

## THE FAUVISTS' ROLE

The artistic movement known as fauvism involved a group of artists at the turn of the 19th and 20th centuries who were protesting conventional forms and were seeking a new means of expression. The artists deviated from a naturalist use of color. Their compositions—such as Henri Matisse's *Woman with a Hat*—deliberately attempted to release color from form. Use of the "wrong" colors by the fauvists is, however, not evidence of color blindness, but

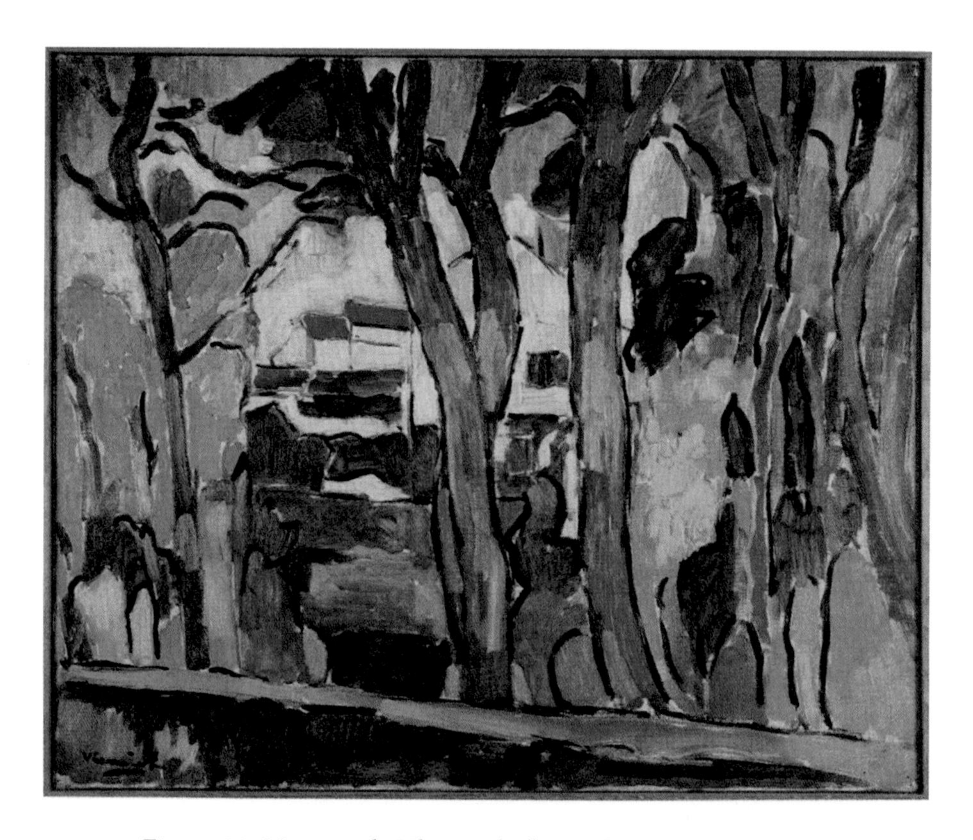

Figure 22. Maurice de Vlaminck: "Les arbres rouges" (1906). Vlaminck belonged to the fauvists, who deliberately used inappropriate colors. Here such colors were not a mark of color blindness, but a means of expression. (Musée National d'Art Moderne, Centre Pompidou, Paris, BONO 2010. Photo RMN).

rather an attempt to release the artist from conventional depictions and allow, as Matisse put it, a more vigorous, emotional and expressive power.

This special way of painting has given us a unique insight into how the brain works. Semir Zeki considers that the fauvists and their followers have been pioneers and purveyors of knowledge about the visual process and color perception in the brain (Zeki 1999). Today we can measure brain activity during different tasks. Zeki observes that when we look at paintings with natural colors the brain activity differs from when we look at images with unnatural colors. Looking at an abstract composition with no shape and no customary colors, as in the style of Piet Mondrian, the activity in the brain is limited to areas V1 and V4. Looking at natural objects or images of "natural "colors, the brain activity connects new and larger areas in the temporal lobe, the memory center (hippocampus), and the frontal lobe.

This shows how art can be related to the science of the brain and color perception.

## DEVIANT COLOR VISION AS AN EXPLANATION

More than physiological contexts must be used when we try to explain the individual character of works of art. Colors kick off a subjective experience explained by other laws. A work of art can be a baffling deviation to some, but may to others a distinctive, enriching experience. Color compositions, the sparkle of the colors chosen, and variations in shades or contrasts can all trigger intense feelings in the individual observer.

The eye is just one among many means of artistic creation. We must avoid letting the discovery of an error in visual perception influence the assessment of the artwork or the artist. Confirmation that the artist is color blind does not justify a negative review any more than a note about Beethoven's deafness would be appropriate to a critique of his music. An artist must be judged solely by his work. Much of a painting's strangeness is not a fault or feature of the artist's eye, but rather is an expression of the artist's ideas and emotions. Art has its own way to go and where you cannot demand explanations—or insist upon an artist's physical deficiencies. The ineffable in art remains ineffable.

# APPENDIX

## GLOSSARY

**Amblyopia:** Reduced vision due to lack of stimulation in young age.

**AMD**= Age related macula degeneration.

**Aphakia**: absence of the lens of the eye.

**Autosomal heredity**: transmitted by ordinary paired chromosomes, not gender based heredity.

**CAD**: "Color Assessment and Diagnosis" ; a new test for identifying colors.

**Chromatic adaptation**: the process when the eye is getting accustomed to a certain color.

**Chromatopsia**: seeing the surroundings tinted in a certain color.

**Chromosome**: Chromatin elements in the nucleus built up by DNA threads carrying the genes.

**Color anomia**: a condition where he individual can see colors, but is not able to understand what he or she is seeing.

**Cool colors:** Colors from the short wavelength part of the spectrum, i.e. blue, violet and blue-green.

**DALTONIANA**: Newsletter of the IRGCV

**DNA** = deoxyribonucleic acid. Protein parts of the chromosomes made up of genes linearly arranged.

**Eclampsia**: Convulsive seizures or coma following development of hypertension and renal failure in pregnancy (Preeclampsia= beginning eclampsia).

**Encephalitis**: inflammation of the brain.

**Fauvism**: term used for a circle of painters characterized by their use of pure, highly contrasting and "wrong" colors. Introduced from 1905. Les fauves (fr)= wild beaches.

**Gene**: the biological unit of heredity; attached to a certain spot (locus) on the chromosome.

**Hemizygotic** heredity: Precence of only one chromosome in a pair of chromosomes, for instance in one X-cromosome in men.

**Heterozygotic**: having different type of gene in paired chromosomes.

**Homozygotic:** having the same type of gene in paired chromosomes.

**ICI** = International Commission on Illumination.

**Interference filter**: Filter transmitting light of one or nearly one wavelength, i.e. producing monochromatic or nearly monochromatic light..

**IRGCV** = International Research Group on Color Vision.

**Køllner's rule**: Lesions of the outer retinal layers causes a blue-yellow defect, while lesions of the inner retinal layers causes a red-green defect.

**Light source C** (of the ICI): the generally accepted locus for "standard white"/ Daylight.

**Low pressure sodium lamp**: Fluorescent tube filled with Na-gas under low pressure. Emits monochromatic light of wavelength. 589 nanometer.

**Monochromacy**: only one color.

**Nanometer (nm):** one billionth of a meter; $1/10^{11}$ meter or $1/10^{8}$ mm

**Nystagmus**: Involuntary, trembling movements of the eyes ("jiggling eyes").

**PAPI**=" Precision approach Path Indicator"; referring to the signal system used in the airports to direct the airplanes during landing.

**Photophobia**: aversion to bright light.

**Pitt's law**: Differential wavelength discrimination in the color defective is best where intrinsic saturation is poorest.

**Prosopagnosia**: Lack of ability to recognize faces

**Pseudo-isochromatic** = apparently the same color. Color charts with figures composed of colors that are regularly confused by people with color vision deficiencies.

**Psychophysical**: measuring procedure based on subjective observations.

**Purkinji shift**: changing from day vision to night vision. (i.e. from vision dominated by cones to rod vision). Maximum sensitivity changing from about 550 nanometer to about 507 nanometer.

**Recessive trait** = yielding manifestation, Heredity not transmitted unless by double dose of genes.

**Scotopic vision** (night vision): vision based on rods only. No perception of color. Maximum sensitivity about 507 nanometer.

**Simultaneous contrast**: when a color provoke impression of another color nearby.

**Synaestesia**: when stimulation of one sense system releases sensations in other sense systems.

**Tint**: weak chromaticity, shade of color.

**Transient tritanopia**: reduction of blue perception in a moment after extinction of a yellow illumination.

**Warm colors**: Colors from the middle and long wavelength part of the spectrum, i.e. yellow-green, yellow, orange and red.

**Xanthopsia**: seeing the surroundings tinted in yellow color..

# ADDITIONAL INDEX OF NAMES

## RESEARCHERS

**Bonnet**, Charles (1720-1793)
Swiss natural scientist and philosoph. His syndrome first described in 1760 (and introduced into English-speaking psychiatry in 1982).

**Cohn**, Hermann (1838-1906)
A leading ophthalmologist in Germany. Founded his separate Eye Clink in Breslau.

**Daae**, Anders (1838-1910)
Practicing physician in Kragerø, Norway; in recent years a prison governor.

**Dalton**, John (1766-1844)
English physicist and Chemist. Founder of the modern atom-theory.
Teacher at The New College in Manchester.

**Donders**, Frans Cornelis (1818-1889)
Professor of ophthalmology at Utrecht.

**Farnsworth**, Dean (1902-1959)
Commander of the United States Navy; attached to The Naval Submarine Research Laboratory in New London.

von **Goethe**, Johann Wolfgang (1749-1832)
German author famous for his lyric poetry and author of Faust. Studied natural science. Introduced a new color theory (1810).

**Hardy**, LeGrand (1895-1954)
U.S. ophthalmologist and scientist; practicing specialist in New York.

von **Helmholtz**, Hermann Ludwig Ferdinand (1821-1894)
Professor of physiology at Kønigsberg, Bonn, Heidelberg and of physics in Berlin.

**Hering**, Ewald (1834-1918)
Physiologist of Vienna, Prague and Leipzig.

**Holmes**, Sir Gordon Morgan (1876-1965)
Neurologist at the National Hospital for Nervous Diseases and at Moorfields Eye Hospital, London.

**Holmgren**, Alaric Frithiof (1831-1897)
Swedish physician and Professor of Physiology.

**Horner**, Johann Friedrich (1831-1886)
Swiss ophthalmologist and professor at the University of Zurich. An independent Eye Clinic was built up by Horner who became its director.

**Ishihara**, Shinobu (1879-1963)
Japanese ophthalmologist and professor at The Imperial University of Tokyo.
The Ishihara Color Vision Test first published in 1917.

**Køllner**, Hans
German ophthalmologist and physiologist; introduced the Køllner's rule (1912).

**Leonardo** da Vinci (1452-1519)
Florentine painter and sculptor besides engineer and scientist: one of the greatest genius in the European culture.

**Liebreich**, Richard L (1830-1917)
German ophthalmologist; published "Atlas der Ophthalmoscopie" 1863.

**Linksz**, Arthur,
Clinical Professor of Ophthalmology, New York.

**Maxwell**, James Clerk (1831-1879)
Professor of experimental physics at Cambridge. The originator of the electro- magnetic theory of light.

**Monge**, Gaspard (1746-1818)
French mathematician. Among founders of the École Polythechnique. Played a central part in the French Revolution.

**Nagel** W A
Professor in Berlin. Developed his anomaloscope in 1907.

**Newton**, Sir Isaac (1642-1727)
English physicist and mathematician. Regarded as the most prominent scientist of all time and a key figure in the scientific revolution. Professor in mathematics at the Cambridge University. President of The Royal Society.

Lord **Rayleigh**, John William Strutt (1842-1919)
Professor of Experimental Physics at the University of Cambridge and Professor of Natural Philosophy at the Royal Institution. Awarded the Nobel Prize 1904.

**Rushton**, William Albert Hugh (1901-1980)
British physiologist; worked at Cambridge University and Florida State University.

**Schiøtz**, Hjalmar August (1850-1927)
Layed the foundation for the eye speciality in Norway and became the first

Norwegian professor of ophthalmology in 1901. A Schiøtz' medal and prize is established by the Norwegian Ophthalmic Society.

**Schiøtz**, Ingolf (1887-1961)
Practicing Ophthalmologist in Oslo; the son of Hjalmar Schiøtz.

**Stengel**, Otto Christiian (1794-1890)
Physician at the Roeros Copper Mining Company, Norway. Gave the first description of Ceroid Lipofuscinosis (1826).

**Stiles**, Walter Stanley (1901-1985)
Scientist at the National Physical Laboratory, Teddington, England.

**Stilling**, Jacob (1842-1915)
German ophthalmologist from Kassel; Titular Professor at the University of Strassburg.

**Velhagen** jun., Karl
Professor of Ophthalmology Stuttgart.

**Verriest**, Guy (1927-1988)
Belgium ophthalmologist and research worker; founder and initiator of the first meeting of the International Research Group on Color Vision Deficiencies (IRGCVD) in Ghent in 1971. Honored by a special award, the Verriest lecture.

**Wald**, George (1906-1997)
Professor of biology at Harvard University. Famous for studies of metabolism of the visual pigments. Was awarded a Nobel Price in 1968.

**Weale**, Robert A.
Professor of Visual Science, Institute of Ophthalmology, University of London.

**Waaler**, Georg Henrik Magnus (1895-1983)
Heredity researcher and expert on forensic medicine. Professor of Forensic Medicine at the Rikshospital, the National Hospital, Oslo.

**Young,** Thomas (1773-1829)
Professor of natural philosophy at the Royal Institution in London.

## ARTISTS

Prince **Eugen,** Napoleon Nicolaus (1865-1947)
Swedish painter, Prince of Sweden. 4th son of King Oscar II.

Van **Gogh**, Vincent (1853-1890)
Dutch painter. Painted from the Netherlands and Belgium and the last years from Arles in the South of France.

**Hammershøi**, Vilhelm (1864-1916)
Danish painter well-known for figurative and architecture compositions.

**Henry**, Paul (1876-1958)
Irish painter with motifs from rustic life, famous for his paintings from the Irish landscapes.

**Homer,** Dodge Martin (1836-1897)
American landscape painter.

von **Jawlensky**, Alexei (1864-1941)
Native Russian; painter with abstract combinations of shapes and colors.

**Léger**, Fernand (1881-1955)
French painter with links to Futurist art.

**Matisse**, Henri (1869-1954)
French painter, leading exponent of the "fauves".

**Meryon,** Charles (1821-1868)
Romantic etcher. Grew up in Paris. Gave up oil-painting and turned to printmaking.

**Messiaen**, Olivier (1908-1992)
French musician and major composer of the 20th century.

**Mondrian**, Piet (1872-1944)
Dutch painter characterized by reduction of form to purely geometrical shapes and only few colors.

**Monet**, Claude (1840-1926)
Exponent of the French impressionists.

**Munch**, Edvard (1863-1944)
Norwegian painter, pioneer of the expressionism.

**Rouault,** George (1871-1958)
French painter.

de **Vlaminck**, Maurice (1876-1958)
French painter linked with the Fauvists.

## REFERENCES

Barbur, J, Evans, S & Milburn, N. *Minimum Color Vision Requirements for Professional Flight Crew. Part III: Recommendations for New Color Vision Standards.* Report, Washington DC 20591: Office of Aerospace Medicine, 2009.

Barbur, John L & Konstantakopoulou, Evgenia. "Changes in color vision with decreasing light level: separating the effects of normal aging from disease." *Journal of the Optical Society of America A*, 2012, 29 ed.: 27-35.

Berg, Kåre. "Fargesynets genetikk (Genetics of color vision)." *Nordisk Medicin*, 1967: 1456-1459.

Birch, Jennifer. «On the worldwide prevalence of red-green colour deficiency.» Redigert av Rigmor C. Baraas. *The 21st Symposium of the International Colour Vision Society.* 2011.

Breslauer Zeitung. *Über Farbenblindheit (About color blindness).* Zentralblatt für praktische Augenheilkunde, 1878, 82-86.

Chapanis, A. "Spectral saturation and its relation to color-vision defects." *Journal of Experimental Psychology*, 1944, 34 ed.: 24.

Charman, W N & Evans, N C. "Possible Effects of Changes in Lens Pigmentation on the Colour Balance of an Artist's Work." *British Journal of Physiological Ophthalmology 32*, 1976, 32 ed.: 23- 31.

Cohn, H. "III Gestickte Buchstaben zur Diagnose der Farbenblindheit (Suppressed letters for diagnosis of color blindness)." *Zentralblatt für praktische Augenheilkunde*, 1878, 2 ed.: 77-78.

Cole, B L & Maddocks, J D. "Defective colour vision is a risk factor in driving." *Colour Vision Deficiencies XIII*, 1997: 471-481.

Daae, Anders. *Farveblindhed og Opdagelse af Farveblinde med Tabel (Color blindness and discovery of color blinds with a table).* Kragerø: Bundis Bogtrykkeri, 1877.

Daae, Anders."Ein Beitrag zur Statistik der Farbenblindheit (A contribution to the statistics of color blindness)." *Zentralblatte für praktische Augenheilkunde*, 1878, 2 ed.: 79.

Dain, S J & Hughes, L E. "Survey of the colour vision demands in fire-fighting." In *Normal and Defective Colour Vision*, edited by J D, Pokorny, J & Knoblauch, K Mollon, 347-353. Oxford: Oxford University Press, 2003.

Damasio, A R & Damasio, H. "Brain and Language." *Scientific American*, 1992, 267 ed.: 63- 71.

Damasio, A, Yamada, T, Damasio, H, Corbett, J, & McKee, J. "Central achromatopsia: behavioral, anatomic and physiologic aspects." *Neurology*, 1980, 30 ed.: 1064- 1071.

Derefeldt, G. *Färg, visuell sökning och begrepsbildning (Color, visual searching and conceptualizing).* Excerpt, Linköping: Försvarets Forskningsanstalt, 1993.

Dietrichs, Espen & Stien, Ragnar. *The Brain and the Arts.* Oslo: Koloritt Forlag, 2008.

Farnsworth, Dean. *What the color defective person sees.* Baltimore: Munsell Color Company, 1951.

Fletcher, Robert J. "Experiences with assisting daltonics." *Documenta Ophthalmologica Proceeding Series*, 1982, 33 ed.: 355-356.

Fletcher, Robert J. "The Fletcher CAM lantern colour vision test." *Clinical*, July 29, 2005: 24-26.

Fletcher, Robert J. "A modified D-15 test." *Modern Problems of Ophthalmology*, 1972, 11 ed.: 22-24.

Francois J, Verriest G. "On Aquired Deficiency of Colour Vision." *Vision Research*, 1961: 201- 219.

Francois, J, Verriest, G, Mortier, V & Vanderdonck, R. "De la fréquence des dyschromatopsies congénitales chez l'homme (About the frequency of congenital dyschromatopsies in human)." *Annales d'oculistique*, 1957, 189 ed.: 5-16.

Gallagher J R & Gallagher, C D. "Color vision screening of preschool and first grade children." *Archives of Ophthalmology*, 1964, 72 ed.: 200-211.

Gibson, H C, Smith D M & Alpern, M. "Specificity in digitoxin toxicity." *Archieves of Ophthalmology*, 1965, 74 ed.: 154-158.

Graham C H, Hsia Y, Berger E. "Luminosity functions for normal and dichromatic subjects including a case of unilateral color blindness." *Journal of Optical Society of America*, 1955: 45, 40, 16.

Green, G J & Lessel, S. "Acquired cerebral dyschromatopsia." *Archives of Ophthalmology*, 1977, 95 ed.: 121-128.

Hansen E, Frøyshov-Larsen, I & Berg, K. "A familial syndrome of progressive cone dystrophy, degenerative liver disease, endocrine dysfunction and hearing defect." *Acta ophthalmologica*, 1976, 54 ed.: 129-144.

Hansen, Egill. "Noen data om Anders Daae og hans farvesansprøve (Some Notes on Anders Daae and his Colour Vision Test)." In *Nordisk Medicinhistorisk Årsbok*, 113-121. 1978.

Hansen, Egill. "Examination of colour vision by use of induced contrast colours." *Acta Ophthalmologica*, 1976, 54 ed.: 611- 22.

Hansen, Egill. "The disturbance of colour vision after sunbathing." *Colour Vision Deficiencies V*, 1980, 5 ed.: 157-161.

Hansen, Egill. *Selective chromatic adaptation studies with special reference to a method combining Stile's two-colour threshold technique and static perimetry.* Oslo: Studentsamskipnaden, 1979. Thesis.

Hem, Erlend. "Fargeblinde leger - er det noe problem? (Color blind doctors - is it a problem?)." *Tidsskrift for den Norske Legeforening*, 2004, 124 ed.: 195-197.

Henmo, Ola. "Mitt liv som fargeblind (My life as a color blind)." *Aftenposten A-Magasinet*, no. 24 (2010): 32-34.

Holm, E & Lodberg, C V. "A family with total colour-blindness." *Acta ophthalmologica*, 1940, 18 ed.: 224-258.

Hunt, D M, Kanwaljit, S D, Bowmaker, J K & Mollon, J D. «The Chemistry of John Dalton's Color Blindness.» *Science*, 1995, 267. utg.: 984-988.

Jaeger, W & Krastel, H. «Colour vision deficiencies caused by pharmacotherapy.» *Colour Vision Deficiencies VIII*, 1987.

Jaeger, Wolfgang. "Die Geschichte der Farbensinn (The history of color vision)." *Klinsche Monatsbletter für Augenheilkunde*, 1994, 205 ed.: 251-254.

Johansen, Otto. *Øyelegekunstens historie i Norge (The history of ophthalmological arts in Norway).* Oslo: Universitetsforlaget, 1978.

Kalmus, H. *Diagnosis and Genetics of defective Colour Vision.* Oxford: Pergamon Press, 1965.

Karpe, Gösta. "Könstnärsögats förvandlingar (Changes in the artist's eye)." *Svenska Dagbladet*, December 1962.

Kinney, J A S, Paulson, H M & Beare A N. "The ability of color defectives to judge signal lights at sea." *Journal of Optical Society of America*, 1979, 69 ed.: 106-113.

Knutsen, J E. "Leketøysoldater og figurer (Toy soldiers and figures)." 2000.

Krill, A E & Fishman, G A. «Aquired color vision defects.» *Transaction of American Academi of Ophthalmology and Otolaryngology*, 1971, 75. utg.: 1095-1111.

Krill, A E, Smith, V C & Pokorny, J. "Similarities between congenital tritan defects and dominant optic-nerve atrophy: Coincidence or identity?" *Journal of Optical Socity of America*, 1970, 60 ed.: 1132- 1139.

Kurtenbach, A, Erb, C, Adler, M & Born, B. "Colour vision in diabetics tested by the Fransworth-Munsell 28-Hue desaturated test." *Color Research and Application. Supplementum Volume*, 2001, 26 ed.: 292-296.

Lanthony, Philippe. "Daltonism in painting." *Color research and application Supplementum Volume*, 2001, 26 ed.: 12-16.

Lanthony, Philippe. *Les yeux des peintres (The painters' eyes).* Lausanne: L'Age d'Homme, 1999.

Larsson, Sven. *Konstnärens öga (The artist's eye).* Stockholm: Natur och Kultur, 1965.

Linksz, Arthur. *An Essay on Color Vision.* New York: Grune & Stratton, 1964.

Mancuso, K, Hauswirth, W W, Li, Q, Connor, T B, Kuchebbecker, J A, Mauck, M C, Neitz, J & Neitz, M. "Gene Therapy for Red-Green Colour Blindness in Adult Primates." *Nature*, September 2009.

Marmor, Michael F & Ravin, James G. *The Artist's Eyes. Vision and the history of art.* New York: Abrams, 2009.

Melander, P. "Grönt fel för synskadade (Green errornous for visually handicapped)." *Dagens nyheter*, October 1997.

Melin, A D, Fedigan, L M, Hiramatsu, C, Sendall, C L & Kawamura, S. "Effects of colour vision phenotype on insect capture." *Animal behaviour*, 2007, 73 ed.: 205-214.

Mollon, J D. «" --aus dreyerley Arten von Membranen oder Molekülen": George Palmer's Legacy.» *Color Vision Deficiencies XIII*, 1997: 3-20.

Mollon, J. "Monge. The Verriest Lecture, Lyon 2005." *Visual Neuroscience*, 2006, 23 ed.: 297-309.

Moreland A B, Kennard C, Lawden M & Ruddock K H. "Visual functions in a patient with acquired achromatopsia." *Documenta Ophthalmologica Proceedings Series*, 1995, 57 ed.: 87- 94.

Neitz, Maureen & Neitz, Jay. "A new mass screening test for color-vision deficiencies in children." *Color Research and Application. Supplementum Volume.*, 2001, 26 ed.: 239- 249.

Nordby, Knut. «Vision in a complete achromat: a personal account.» I *Night Vision*, av R F, Sharpe, L T and Nordby, K Hess, redigert av R F, Sharpe, L T & Nordby, K Hess, 290-315. Cambridge: Cambridge University Press, 1990.

Ogata, A, Tohgo, S, Kawatsu, M, Kawahira, K & Tanaka, N. "Central achromatopsia, associative visual agnosia, and prosopagnosia due to fusiform gyrus infarction." Case report, 2005.

Oliphant, D and Hovis, J K. "Comparison of the D-15 and City University (second) color vision tests." *Vision Research*, 1998, 38 ed.: 3461-3465.

Pickford, R W. "Individual Differences in Colour Vision." By Routledge and Kegan Paul. London, 1951.

Pickford, R W. "The Genetics of Colour Blindness." In *Colour Vision*, by R W Pickford. London: Reuck & Knight, 1965.

Pickford, R W. "Compound hemizygotes for red-green colour vision defects." *Vision Research*, 1962, 2 ed.: 245-252.

Pokorny, J, Smith, V C, Verriest, G & Pinckers A. *Congenital and Acquired Color Vision Defects.* New York: Grune & Stratton Inc, 1979.

Ramachandran, V S and Blakeslee, Sandra. *Phantoms in the Brain.* London: Harper Perennial, 2005.

Ramachandran, V S. *The Tall-Tale Brain.* New York: W. W. Norton & Company, 2011.

Sacks, Oliver. *Musicophilia. Tales of music and the brain.* New York: Alfred A. Knopf. Inc., 2007.

Sacks, Oliver. "The Case of the Colorblind Painter." In *An Anthropologist on Mars*, by Oliver Sacks, edited by Oliver Sacks, 3-41. New York: Vintage Books, 1995.

Sacks, Oliver. *The Island of the Colourblind and Cycad Island.* New York: Alfred A. Knopf, Inc, 1996.

Sacks, Oliver. *The Mind's Eye.* Edited by Oliver Sacks. New York: Alfred A. Knopf, 2010.

Sällström, Pehr. *Färgblindas miljöupplevelse (Environmental consciousness of the color blind).* Stockholm: KTH, 1978.

Seim, Thorstein & Valberg, Arne. "Image diffusion in cataracts affects chromatic and achromatic contrast perception differently." *Documenta Ophthalmologica Proceeding Series*, 1993, 56 ed.: 153-161.

Sharpe, L T & Jägle, H. "Ergonomic consequences of dichromacy." *Color Research and Application. Supplumentum Volume*, 2001, 26 ed.: 269- 272.

Spalding, J. "Doctors with inherited colour vision deficiency: their difficulties in clinical work." *Colour Vision Deficiencies XIII*, 1997: 483-489.

Sperling, H G. «Blue receptor distribution in primates from intense light and histochemical studies.» *Colour Vision Deficiencies V*, 1980: 30-44.

Spitalny, I A, Devoe, J B & Fenske, H D. "Color perception in unilateral aphakia." *Archives of Ophthalmology*, 1969, 82 ed.: 592-595.

Stengel, Otto Christian. "Beretning om et mærkeligt Sygdomstilfælde hos fire Søskende i Nærheden af Røraas (Account of a singular Illness among four Siblings in the Vicinity of Røraas)." *EYR - et medicinsk Tidsskrift*, 1826, 1 ed.: 347-352.

Stiles, W S. "Increment thresholds & the mechanisms of colour vision." *Documenta Ophthalmologica*, 1949, 3 ed.: 138-163.

Stilling, J. *Die Prüfung des Farbensinnes beim Eisenbahn- und Marinenpersonal. Tafeln zur Bestimmung der Rot-Grünblindheit (Examination of color vision of railway- and navy personell. Plates for diagnosing red-green blindness)* . Cassel: Theodor Fischer, 1878.

*The 20th-Century Art Book.* London: Phaidon Press Limited, 1999.

The Norwegian Registry of Blindness. *Blindness and partial sightedness in Norway.* Report, Oslo: The Ministry of Health, 1995.

Trevor-Roper, P D. "The influence of eye disease on pictorial art." *Proceedings of Royal Society of Medicine (Ophthalmology)*, 1959, 52 ed.: 721-744.

Velhagen, K. *Pflügerhaken-Tafeln zur Prüfung des Farbensinnes (Plow-hook Charts for Examening the Color Vision).* Leipzig: VEB Georg Thieme, 1980.

Verhulst, S & Maes, F W. "Scotopic vision in colour-blinds." *Vision Research*, 1998, 38 ed.: 3387-3390.

Verriest, Guy. "L'influence de l'âge sur les fonctions visuelles de l'homme (Influence of age on the visual functions in man)." *Bulletin de l'A̍cademie Royale de Medicine*, 1971, 11 ed.: 527-577.

Verriest, Guy. "Further studies on acquired deficiency of color discrimination." *Journal of Optical Society of America*, 1963, 53 ed.: 185-195.

Verriest, Guy. *Recent advances in the study of the acquired deficiencies of colour vision.* Firenze: Fondazione "Giorgio Ronchi", 1974.

Vingrys, A J & Cole. B L. "Are color vision standards justified for the transport industry?" *Ophthalmic Physiological Optics*, 1988, 8 ed.: 257-274.

Vos, J J & Walraven, P L. "On the deviation of the foveal receptor primaries." *Vision Research* , 1971, 2 ed.: 799-818.

Waaler, George H M. "Über die Erbliichkeitsverhältnisse der vershiedenen Arten von angeborener Rotgrünblindheit (About the hereditary relationship of the different types of congenital red-green blindness)." *Zeitschrift für induktive Abstammungs- und Vererbungslehre*, 1927, 45 ed.: 279-333.

Zeki, Semir. "Colour Coding in Rhesus Monkey Prestriate Cortex." *Brain Research*, 1973, 53 ed.: 422-427.

Zeki, Semir. *Inner Vision.* New York: Oxford University Press Inc., 1999.

Zihl, J. *Colour vision deficits in Rehabilitation of Visual Disorders after Brain Injury.* Edited by J Zihl. Psychology Press Ltd, 2000.

## GENERAL INDEX

Made in the USA
Middletown, DE
31 August 2018